WORLD BANK WORKING PAPER NO. 68

HIV/AIDS in the Western Balkans

Priorities for Early Prevention in a High-Risk Environment

Joana Godinho
Nedim Jaganjac
Dorothee Eckertz
Adrian Renton
Thomas Novotny
Lisa Garbus

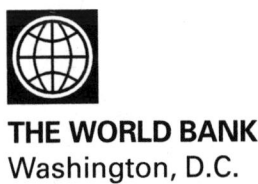

THE WORLD BANK
Washington, D.C.

ISBN-10: 0-8213-6394-8   ISBN-13: 978-0-8213-6394-2
eISBN: 0-8213-6395-6
ISSN: 1726-5878   DOI: 10.1596/978-0-8213-6394-2

Joana Godinho is a Senior Health Specialist at the World Bank. Nedim Jaganjac and Dorothee Eckertz are Health Specialists at the World Bank. Adrian Renton is a Professor of Epidemiology at the Imperial College, London. Thomas Novotny is a Professor of International Health at the University of California in San Francisco. Lisa Garbus is a Senior Researcher at the University of California in San Francisco.

Photo by David Seban, Médecin du Monde: Rave Party in the Balkans

Library of Congress Cataloging-in-Publication Data

HIV/AIDS in the western Balkans : priorities for early prevention in a high-risk environment / Joana Godinho [et al.].
   p. cm. – (World Bank working paper; no. 68)
Includes bibliographical references.
ISBN-13: 978-0-8213-6394-2
ISBN-10: 0-8213-6394-8
   I. HIV infection–Balkan Peninsula. 2. AIDS (Disease)–Balkan Peninsula. I. Godinho, Joana. 11951-II. Series.

RA643.86.A783H555 2005
362.196'9792'009496–dc22   2005053846

Contents

LIST OF TABLES

List of Figures

List of Boxes

Acknowledgments

This study was prepared by a team led by Joana Godinho, which included Nedim Jaganjac, Dorothee Eckertz, Adrian Renton, Thomas Novotny, and Lisa Garbus.[1] The background paper on HIV/AIDS and STIs was based on country reports prepared by Eduard Kakarriqi (Albania), Semra Cavaljuga (Bosnia and Herzegovina), Skender Syla, Xhevat Jakupi (Kosovo), Elisaveta Stikova, Zarko Karadzovski (Macedonia), Boban Mugosa (Montenegro), Danijela Simic, Gordana Rajin, Milan Bjekic (Serbia), and Jim Chauvin (Canadian Public Health Association—CPHA). George Shakarishvili and Linda Currie edited the first draft of the study report. Julie Wagshal, Gizella Diaz, Carmen Laurente, and Anahit Poghosyan prepared the paper for distribution and printing in English. Mirjana Karahasanovic, Mirjana Popovic, Rajna Cemerska, Marina Petrovic, and Florian Tomini organized a GDLN Videoconference to discuss the study main findings and recommendations, and assisted the preparation of the study for printing in Albanian, Bosnian-Croatian, Macedonian, and Serbian. Stuart Tucker prepared the study for printing in English.

The study team is grateful to the Ministries of Health, Justice, Internal Affairs and Finances; National AIDS Committees and/or Programs; as well as to all NGOs and regional partners that provided data and participated in meetings and a GDLN videoconference to discuss the main issues identified in Albania, Bosnia and Herzegovina, Kosovo, Macedonia, and Serbia and Montenegro, and study recommendations. The study benefited from comments from Silva Bino, Klodian Rjepaj, Holba Koci, Erion Basho, Arian Boci, Ardian Paravami and Genc Mucollari from Albania; Zeljka Mudrovic, Zlatko Cardaklija, Radovan Bratic, Jasna Sadic, Zehra Dizdarevic, Jelena Ravlija, Bakir Nakas, and Michael Boynton from Bosnia and Herzegovina; Ivana Misic, Danijela Simic and Boban Mugosa from Serbia and Montenegro; Shpend Elezi, Isuf Dedushaj, Edone Deva and Fatime Qosaj from Kosovo; Snezana Cicevalieva, Vesna Veljic-Stefanovska and Vladanka Andreeva from Macedonia; Eduard Petruscu, Jadranka Mimica, Vladanka Andreeva and Ranko Perovic, from UNAIDS; Deborah McWhiney, Alketa Zazo, Sanja Memisevic, Jill Zarclin and Kerry Neal, from UNICEF; and Vladimir Lazarevik, from Project Hope.

The study team is also thankful to the study Peer Reviewers—Henning Mikkelsen from UNAIDS; Jim Chauvin, from the Canadian Public Health Association; Michael Borowitz, from the Soros Foundation, and Patricio Marquez, from the World Bank, for their helpful insights. In addition Jonathan Brown, from the Global AIDS Unit at the World Bank; Kanthan Shankar, World Bank Manager in Kosovo; Nancy Cooke, Lead Country Officer; Merrell J. Tuck-Primdahl and Mario Bravo, from the External Department;

---

1. Joana Godinho is a Senior Health Specialist at the World Bank. Nedim Jaganjac is a Health Specialist at the World Bank. Dorothee Eckertz is a Health Specialist at the World Bank. Adrian Renton is a Professor of Epidemiology at the Imperial College, London. Thomas Novotny is a Professor of International Health at the University of California in San Francisco. Lisa Garbus is a Senior Researcher at the University of California in San Francisco.

Gloria La Cava, from the Social Development Department; Armin Fidler, Health Sector Manager; Betty Hanan, Monika Huppi and numerous other colleagues from the Human Development Network at the World Bank provided useful comments.

The World Bank		
Vice President	:	Shigeo Katsu
Country Director	:	Orsalia Kalantzopoulos
Sector Director	:	Charles Griffin
Sector Manager	:	Armin Fidler
Task Team Leader	:	Joana Godinho

Acronyms and Abbreviations

APHEW	Aids Foundation East-West
AIDS	Acquired Immune Deficiency Syndrome
ARV	Antiretroviral
CA	Central Asia
CAR	Central Asia Republics
CCM	Country Coordination Mechanism
CDC	Centers for Disease Control and Prevention
CEE	Central and Eastern Europe
CIDA	Canadian International Development Agency
CPHA	Canadian Public Health Association
CSW	Commercial Sex Worker
DFA	Direct Fluorescent Assay
DFID	Department for International Development
DOTS	TB Directly Observed Therapy Short-Course
ECA	Europe and Central Asia
ECA/EXT	Europe and Central Asia, External Affairs
ECAVP	Europe and Central Asia, Office of the Vice President
ELISA	Enzyme Linked Immunoabsorbant Assay
EU	European Union
ESCM	Electronic Surveillance Case-Based Management System
FBiH	Federation of Bosnia and Herzegovina
FM	Family Medicine
FSU	Former Soviet Union
FPG	Family Practice Group
GAR	Groups at Risk
GDF	Global Drug Facility
GDP	Gross Domestic Product
GFATM	Global Fund to Fight AIDS, TB and Malaria
GDP	Gross Domestic Product
HBV	Hepatitis B
HFA	Health for All
HIV	Human Immunodeficiency Virus
HR	Harm Reduction
IA	Institutional Assessment
IC	Imperial College, University of London
IDA	International Development Association
IDU	Intravenous Drug User
IDP	Internally Displaced People
IEC	Information, Education and Communication Campaign
IFRC	International Federation of Red Cross
IFT	Indirect Fluorescent Assay
IPH	Institute of Public Health
IHRD	International Harm Reduction Network

IHRP	International Harm Reduction Program
IO	International Organizations
IOM	International Organization for Migration
IPPF	International Planned Parenthood Federation
IUATLD	International Union Against Tuberculosis and Lung Disease
JICA	Japan International Cooperation Agency
KAP	Knowledge, Attitudes and Practices
KfW	German Development Bank (Kreditanstalt für Wiederaufbau)
MDGs	Millennium Development Goals
MDRTB	Multi-Drug Resistant Tuberculosis
MMR	Mass Miniature Radiography (fluorography)
MOH	Ministry of Health
MOIA	Ministry of Internal Affairs
MOJ	Ministry of Justice
MRT	Methadone Replacement Therapy
MSF	Médecins Sans Frontières
MSM	Men who have sex with men
MTCT	Mother to Child Transmission of HIV/AIDS
NGO	Non Governmental Organizations
NTP	National Tuberculosis Program
OECD	Organization for Economic Cooperation and Development
OSI	Open Society Institute
PCR	Polymerase Chain Reaction
PHC	Primary Health Care
PLWHA	People Living with HIV/AIDS
PRM	Participatory Resource Mapping
PSI	Population Services International
RAC	Republican AIDS Commission (of Serbia, of Montenegro)
RAR	Rapid Assessment Response
RDU	Registered Drug User
RM	World Bank Resident Mission
SA	Stakeholder Analysis
SEE	Southeastern European
STI	Sexually-transmitted Infection
SW	Sex worker
TB	Tuberculosis
TG	UN AIDS Thematic Group
UNAIDS	Joint United Nations Program on HIV/AIDS
UNDP	United Nations Development Program
UNFPA	United Nations Fund for Population Assistance
UNGASS	United Nations General Assembly Special Session
UNHCR	UN High Commission on Refugees
UNICEF	United Nations International Children's Fund
UNODC	UN Office for Drug Control and Crime Prevention
USAID	United States Agency for International Development

VCT	Voluntary testing and counseling
WHO	World Health Organization

Executive Summary

This Study was undertaken to enable regional decisionmakers and Bank management to agree on the priorities for early action in the Western Balkans to prevent the spread of HIV/AIDS—and its potential human and economic costs—in the framework of the UN "Three Ones": one national AIDS Strategy that drives alignment of all partners; one national AIDS authority to coordinate it; and one nationally-owned monitoring and evaluation system.

The study also aimed at informing the Bank's policy dialogue and operational work to control HIV/AIDS in the Balkans; and contributing to building up the regional partnership between Governments, civil society, UN agencies, and multilateral and bilateral agencies to prevent HIV/AIDS, sexually-transmitted infections and TB; and to improve public health in this region.

In recent years, Europe and Central Asia (ECA) has seen the world's fastest growing HIV/AIDS epidemic. In Southeastern Europe, reported prevalence of HIV is generally low (Novotny, Haazen, and Adeyi 2003). The Balkans countries under study[2] have reported over 2,000 HIV/AIDS cases since the beginning of the epidemic in 1985. Presently, these countries have a prevalence rate under 0.1 percent, which ranks them among low prevalence countries. This study shows that this may be partly due to a low level of infection among the population; partly a result of inadequate coverage and inaccuracy of surveillance systems, as contextual factors that increase the vulnerability to HIV/AIDS are present in all countries.

The most striking feature in the Balkans is the high-risk environment. All major factors that could serve as contributing factors for the breakout of an HIV/AIDS epidemic are present in the Balkans. Severe political instability, wars and consequent economic crisis and migration in this region over the last 10 years have generated poverty and presented overwhelming challenges which have affected all countries to varying degrees. These factors have also generated the structural conditions necessary to drive the very types of risk behavior and cultural shifts that create vulnerability to HIV and sexually-transmitted infections (STIs), including growth of injecting drug use; commercial sex work and migration; as well as breakdown of traditional family relationships and mores. At the same time, these countries have been making the transition from public health, education and welfare systems which were cast within the socialist mould; and endeavoring to reform these in the face of drastically reduced resource inputs to these systems.

In ECA, HIV/AIDS disproportionably affects youth, eroding a country's human capital— 80 percent of HIV infected people are 30 years old or younger. Most of these countries have very young populations, which have been affected by the process of social transition, wars, unemployment and other factors. Among youth, there is generalized use of drugs and sexual risk behavior. Therefore, the number of cases of HIV has been increasing, especially in Serbia, and incidence of hepatitis C has clearly increased, which suggests that sharing of infected needles is practiced by injecting drug users (IDUs).

---

2. The Balkans countries and territories covered by this study are Albania, Bosnia and Herzegovina, Macedonia, Serbia and Montenegro, and the UN-administered territory of Kosovo.

This study has confirmed that the Balkans region faces a triple jeopardy:

- All structural factors are present to drive epidemics of injecting drug use, followed by generalization through self sustaining epidemics characterized, predominantly, by heterosexual transmission;
- Conflict and economic decline handicap the ability of governments and civil society to make an effective response; and
- Old ideologies and vested interests are set against key elements of intervention known to be effective. An urgent, large and concerted response is required if the effects of these events are not to be felt over many years to come, through a substantial HIV/AIDS epidemic.

Although the low number of cases identified, and lack of reliability of existing data, do not allow to predict with certainty future trends of the HIV/AIDS epidemic in the Balkans, a potential epidemic may develop or be halted in one of three ways:

- Following the pattern of the epidemic in other regional countries, it becomes clearly concentrated on IDUs in the near future, until eventually it spreads to other groups of the population through sexual contact;
- Injecting drug use does not become widespread, and sexual transmission continues to be the most likely route of transmission of the infection and establishment of the epidemic; or
- An epidemic is prevented through early concerted efforts of public sector, NGOs, and the international community in close cooperation with young people at high risk of being infected or that are already infected. In this scenario, highly vulnerable groups reduce the harm of injecting drugs by avoiding associated risky practices such as sharing needles and syringes; and both highly vulnerable groups and vulnerable groups such as youth increase their knowledge about the epidemic and adopt safe sex practices.

Apart from human suffering, an HIV/AIDS epidemic can have a significant impact on costs of care for individuals, households, health services and society as a whole. The Bank has conducted several studies of the potential epidemiological and economic impact of the epidemic. In ECA, these studies were carried out in Belarus, Moldova, Russian Federation and, more recently, in Central Asia (Lundberg 2001; Ruhel and others 2002; Godinho and others 2005). These studies have shown that, in what concerns the economic impact, uninhibited spread of HIV would diminish the economy's long-term growth rate, taking off in Russia an estimated half a percentage point annually by 2010 and a full percentage point annually by 2020.

The epidemic in ECA is still at the early stages, which means that timely, effective interventions can halt and reverse it. All Balkans countries have already started taking action to prevent and control HIV/AIDS, by preparing strategies and raising funding to implement those strategies. However, in addition to significant vulnerability among youth, this study has found weak public health systems and gaps in financing and institutional capacity necessary to implement evidence-based and cost-effective HIV/AIDS Strategies.

Main Issues

The main issues identified by the Study were the following:

- Although all countries, with the exception of Montenegro, have approved HIV/AIDS Strategies prepared with UNAIDS and other partner organizations' assistance, the degree of political commitment to implement the Strategies varies from country to country;
- Most Governments have not yet made specific allocations for HIV/AIDS prevention;
- All countries have applied for funding from the Global Fund Against HIV/AIDS, TB and Malaria, but Albania, Bosnia and Herzegovina, Montenegro and Kosovo have not yet been awarded grants;
- In addition, other international aid has been decreasing in this region, as demand has been rising elsewhere (Africa, Afghanistan, Iraq);
- Information about the most vulnerable groups,[3] including data about knowledge and practices, is scant. Routine surveillance does not provide relevant data, and behavioral and sentinel surveillance of HIV/AIDS and STIs have not yet been established throughout the region;
- Knowledge about the epidemic is very low among most vulnerable groups and the general population;
- Practices reported by the most vulnerable groups, such as sharing of needles and unsafe sex, involve a high risk of infection;
- Epidemic drivers such as trafficking of women and drugs, drug use and commercial sex work put youth at increased risk;
- Public health services in these countries are under-funded and have low capacity, and therefore do not fulfill key public health functions such as policy development, surveillance and prevention including of HIV/AIDS;
- The most vulnerable groups (IDUs, commercial sex workers and others) have only been covered by pilot projects in most countries. For example, although there is higher incidence of HIV/AIDS among sailors and tourist workers in Montenegro, prevention activities targeted specifically at these groups have not yet been developed; and
- Countries that have allocated funding for treatment, such as Macedonia and Serbia, are only able to cover a small number of patients.

Decreasing the risk of an HIV/AIDS epidemic spreading throughout the Balkans region, and becoming a long-term development problem as it has happened in other regions, requires a mix of interventions aimed at reducing the risk of infection in the short term, and interventions aimed at tackling structural factors in the medium to long term. However, it is necessary that political commitment increase for action to occur promptly.

---

3. Highly vulnerable groups include injecting drug users, commercial sex workers, trafficked people, men who have sex with men and prisoners. Other vulnerable groups include migrants, soldiers and peace-keeping forces and other mobile populations.

Prevention interventions are cost-effective and, in the short term, affordable with own-country resources. Medium- and long-term interventions would require donor assistance, including financing by the World Bank. Activities in the short term would aim at ensuring the implementation of approved strategies for prevention of HIV/AIDS; improving the quantity, quality and use of the information available; and covering the most vulnerable groups with harm reduction and safe sex programs. The sustainability of these actions requires improvement of public health services in the medium term. Longer-term interventions would aim at preventing poverty, exclusion and unemployment, for example, by empowering young people to participate in the regional and global labor market.

Key Actions

The recommended key actions for the short and medium term are the following:

Actions for the Short Term

- Implement approved HIV/AIDS Strategies;
- Improve leadership and decision making capacity of national coordination bodies;
- Fund-raise and allocate budgetary funds for HIV/AIDS prevention;
- Establish behavioral and sentinel surveillance throughout the region;
- Inform and educate young people, especially the most vulnerable groups;
- Scale up coverage of most vulnerable groups such as injecting drug users, commercial sex workers, men who have sex with men, sailors, tourist and seasonal workers, and migrants with harm reduction and safe sex programs;
- Adopt evidence-based policies for treatment of people living with HIV/AIDS; and
- Adopt policies on financing, procurement and use of antiretroviral drugs for treatment of people living with HIV/AIDS.

Actions for the Medium and Long Term

- Invest on public health services to enable these to perform key public health functions such as policy development, surveillance and prevention including of HIV/AIDS; and which ensure the sustainability of actions taken in the shorter term; and
- Improve opportunities for young people that decrease risks associated with epidemic drivers such as unemployment, trafficking of people and drugs, use of drugs and commercial sex work; and enable young people to participate in the regional and global labor market.

Specific Actions for Countries and Territories Under Study

Recommendations for priority actions for early prevention of HIV/AIDS in each country or territory under study are highlighted in Table 1. The majority of the proposed actions are similar in all countries, with a few variations according to the specific situation in each country.

Table 1. Specific Actions for Countries and Territories Under Study

	Albania
Funding	▓ Re-submit proposal to the GFATM
	▓ Improve donor coordination
Policy & Intersectoral Coordination	▓ Invest on one multisectoral coordination mechanism
	▓ Implement AIDS Strategy
	▓ Implement anti-trafficking and CSW prevention policies
Surveillance & Institutional Development	▓ Strengthen key public health functions at the IPH (policy, surveillance, health promotion, disease prevention)
	▓ Develop second generation surveillance system
	▓ Build technical capacity in surveillance
Prevention	▓ Improve drug and sex education
	▓ Increase awareness regarding HIV counseling and testing among high risk groups (CSW, migrants, youth)
	▓ Scale up harm reduction programs for IDUs
	▓ Implement youth-targeted programs on income generation, skills development, education and sports
	Bosnia and Herzegovina
Funding	▓ Re-submit proposal to the GFATM
	▓ Mobilize donors and improve donor coordination
Policy & Intersectoral Coordination	▓ Strengthen the multisectoral coordination mechanism
	▓ Integrate AIDS Strategy into Poverty Reduction Strategy
Surveillance & Institutional Development	▓ Strengthen key public health functions at the IPH (policy, surveillance, health promotion, disease prevention)
	▓ Develop second generation surveillance system
	▓ Build technical capacity in surveillance
Prevention	▓ Improve drug and sex education
	▓ Increase awareness of HIV counseling and testing among high risk groups (CSW, mobile population, youth)
	▓ Implement youth-targeted programs on income generation, skills development, education and sports
	Macedonia
Funding	▓ Ensure successful implementation of GFATM grant
	▓ Support NGOs providing HIV/AIDS prevention services
	▓ Raise funds for the medium to longer term
Policy & Intersectoral Coordination	▓ Strengthen the National Multisectoral Commission
	▓ Integrate AIDS Strategy into the national MDGs agenda
	▓ Establish mechanisms for transferring funds to NGOs
Surveillance & Institutional Development	▓ Support management of GFATM grant
	▓ Strengthen key public health functions at the IPH (policy, surveillance, health promotion, disease prevention)
	▓ Develop second generation surveillance system
	▓ Build technical capacity in surveillance

(continued)

Table 1. Specific Actions for Countries and Territories Under Study (*Continued*)

	▨ Strengthen epidemiological and statistical skills at the Medical Faculty and the Institute for Health Protection.
	▨ Strengthen VCT and confidentiality of testing
Prevention	▨ Improve drug and sex education
	▨ Increase awareness of HIV counseling and testing among high risk groups (CSW, drug users, youth)
	▨ Establish harm reduction programs for IDUs
Treatment	▨ Develop policy on use of ARV drugs
Serbia	
Funding	▨ Ensure appropriate implementation of GFATM grant
	▨ Support NGOs providing HIV/AIDS prevention services
	▨ Coordinate implementation of GFATM and DFID grants
	▨ Raise funds for the medium to longer term
Policy & Intersectoral Coordination	▨ Invest on RAC as the multisectoral coordination mechanism
	▨ Establish mechanisms for transferring funds to NGOs
Surveillance & Institutional Development	▨ Develop second generation surveillance
	▨ Build technical capacity in surveillance
	▨ Strengthen key public health functions at the IPH (policy, surveillance, health promotion, disease prevention)
	▨ Initiate Country Response Information System
	▨ Set a system for M&E of response to HIV/AIDS
Prevention	▨ Improve drug and sex education
	▨ Increase awareness of HIV counseling and testing among high risk groups (IDUs, CSWs, migrants, youth)
Treatment	▨ Implement youth-targeted programs on income generation, skills development, education and sports
	▨ Develop policy on use of ARV drugs
Montenegro	
Funding	▨ Re-submit realistic proposal to the GFATM
Policy & Intersectoral Coordination	▨ Invest on RAC as the multisectoral coordination mechanism
	▨ Approve appropriate AIDS Strategy
	▨ Legalize anonymous testing for HIV/AIDS
Surveillance & Institutional Development	▨ Strengthen key public health functions at the IPH (policy, surveillance, health promotion, disease prevention)
	▨ Strengthen second generation surveillance system
	▨ Initiate Country Response Information System
	▨ Build technical capacity in surveillance
Prevention	▨ Improve drug and sex education
	▨ Increase awareness of HIV counseling and testing among high risk groups (sailors, tourist workers, CSW, migrants, youth)
	▨ Establish harm reduction programs for IDUs
	▨ Implement youth-targeted programs on income generation, skills development, education and sports

Table 1. **Specific Actions for Countries and Territories Under Study (*Continued*)**

	Kosovo
Funding	▨ Re-submit proposal to the GFATM
	▨ Improve donor coordination
Policy & Intersec-toral Coordination	▨ Strengthen Kosovo AIDS Commission
	▨ Develop post-conflict trafficking and CSW prevention policies
Surveillance & Institutional Development	▨ Strengthen key public health functions at the IPH
	▨ Strengthen second generation surveillance system
	▨ Build technical capacity in surveillance
Prevention	▨ Improve drug and sex education
	▨ Increase awareness of HIV counseling and testing among high risk groups (CSW, mobile population, youth)
	▨ Establish harm reduction programs for IDUs
	▨ Implement youth-targeted programs on income generation, skills development, education and sports

The World Bank's Role in the Western Balkans

The Bank has had a significant role in prevention and control of HIV/AIDS, being one of the main sources of financing to fight the epidemic globally. The Bank is uniquely positioned to act simultaneously on risk factors and epidemic drivers that require short and longer-term actions.

In the Western Balkans, the Bank will continue to closely monitor the evolution of the HIV/AIDS epidemic. This evidence would inform Bank policy dialogue about AIDS in the region, and the development of Country Partnership and Poverty Reduction Strategies.

Taking into account that international aid is fading out in some of these countries; existing gaps in financing and technical assistance; and that sustainability of the Global Fund to Fight AIDS, TB and Malaria (GFATM) grants is uncertain in the medium term, the Western Balkans Governments and the Bank may want to consider to:

▨ Increase policy dialogue on prevention and control of HIV/AIDS and other communicable diseases such as STIs and tuberculosis; public health functions; and youth vulnerability;

▨ Continue sector work on HIV/AIDS and STIs in the region in cooperation with partner organizations;

▨ Provide leadership training, increased awareness of evidence-based approaches to HIV/AIDS, and technical skills to country counterparts through the World Bank Institute's Leadership Program on AIDS (LPA); and

▨ Invest on AIDS prevention and control:

  i. As part of poverty and sector operations;

ii. On operations that focus on decreasing youth vulnerability and improving public health functions that are key to prevent and control HIV/AIDS. Lessons learned from the proposed Kosovo Youth Development Post-Conflict Grant, which includes HIV/AIDS activities, may be valuable for the development of similar operations in a larger scale in other countries; and

iii. Develop a Regional Strategy for prevention and control of HIV/AIDS that, similarly to a regional operation in Central Asia would be co-financed by grants from IDA and partner organizations active on HIV/AIDS in the Western Balkans.

CHAPTER 1

Introduction

The AIDS pandemic has entered its third decade worldwide, being the fourth most important cause of death globally. HIV/AIDS killed more than 3.1 million people in 2004, and an estimated 4.9 million acquired the human immunodeficiency virus (HIV)—bringing to 39.4 million the number of people living with the virus around the world (UNAIDS 2003a). In Sub-Saharan Africa, HIV/AIDS is now the leading cause of death and the fourth biggest killer globally. Life expectancy has been cut by more than 10 years due to HIV/AIDS infection in several countries. The increasing speed of the spread of the epidemic increases the importance of the problem. Current projections suggest that an additional 45 million people will become infected with HIV in 126 low- and middle-income countries (currently with concentrated or generalized epidemics) between 2002 and 2010, unless the world succeeds in mounting a drastically expanded, global prevention effort.

The acquired immunodeficiency syndrome (AIDS) is caused by the human immunodeficiency virus (HIV), which progressively destroys the body's ability to fight infections and certain cancers. Therefore, AIDS patients may get opportunistic infections. HIV is spread most commonly by having unprotected sex with an infected partner, but it also spreads through contact with infected blood. Because of blood screening and heat treatment, the risk of getting HIV from blood transfusions is extremely small. HIV is frequently spread among injection drug users by sharing needles or syringes contaminated with infected blood. Women can transmit HIV to their babies during pregnancy or birth, or through breast milk.[4]

---

4. NIH website 2003.

Figure 1. HIV—Recent Changes in HIV/AIDS Prevalence

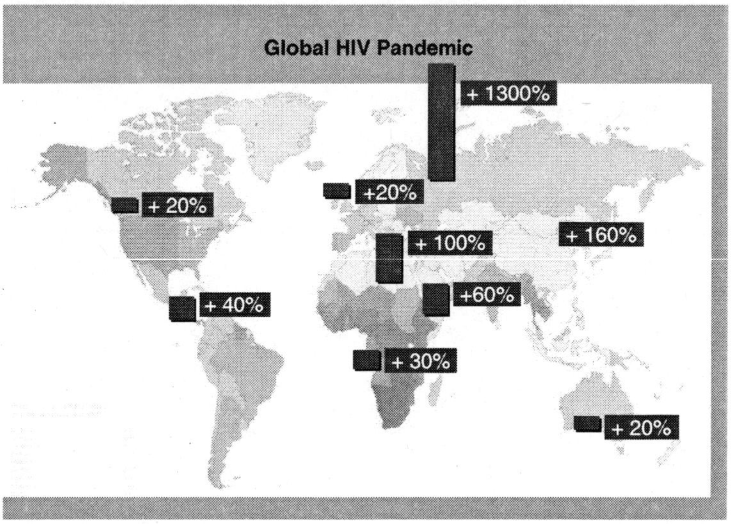

Source: UNAIDS, 2002.

HIV/AIDS mainly affects young people, and spreads quickly in highly vulnerable groups—in ECA, these are injecting drugs users, commercial sex workers, and prisoners. People who are infected with HIV may remain infectious for many years without knowing their status. HIV/AIDS imposes great costs on families and the health system, breaks social cohesion, and reduces life expectancy. There is no vaccine or cure for HIV/AIDS, although antiretroviral drugs, which can be given to newly infected people as well as to AIDS patients, have been a major factor in significantly reducing the number of deaths from AIDS.

HIV/AIDS in ECA

The Region Has the Fastest Growing Rates of HIV Infection in the World

In recent years, ECA has seen the world's fastest growing HIV/AIDS epidemic due to a sharp increase in injecting drug use (IDU). UNAIDS reports 1,300 percent increase in HIV incidence in the region between 1996 and 2001. Officially, the number of HIV infections in ECA has grown from less than 30,000 cases in 1995 to an estimated 1.4 million by the end of 2004; however, the real number is estimated to be much higher. AIDS claimed an estimated 60,000 lives and some 210,000 people were newly infected in 2003. The vast majority of reported infections are among young people, mainly among injecting drug users (IDUs). The major difference between the HIV epidemic in ECA and other regions is the predominant role of drug-injections in HIV transmission.

Figure 2. Growth Rate of Newly Diagnosed HIV Infections in the European Region 1993–2000

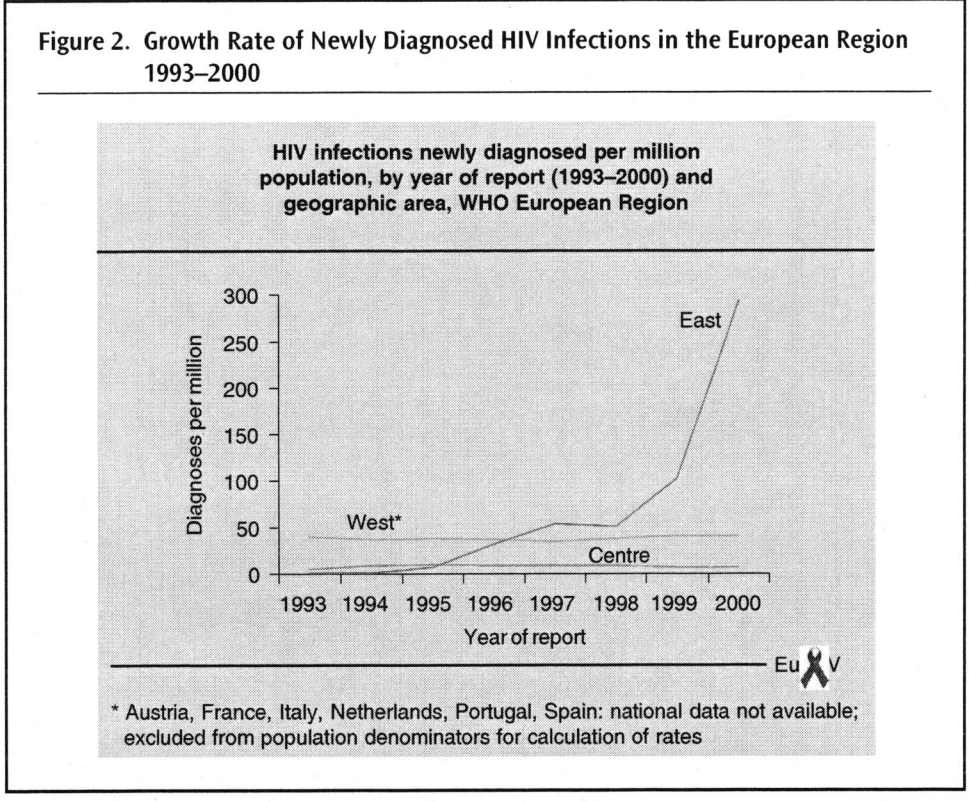

HIV infections newly diagnosed per million population, by year of report (1993–2000) and geographic area, WHO European Region

* Austria, France, Italy, Netherlands, Portugal, Spain: national data not available; excluded from population denominators for calculation of rates

Source: EuroHIV 2003.

The HIV/AIDS Epidemic Has Reached Alarming Levels in ECA

The Russian Federation and Ukraine remain at the vanguard of the HIV/AIDS epidemic in ECA, but many other countries are now experiencing rapidly emerging epidemics. Except for isolated epidemics in the early 1990s related to injecting drug use in Poland, and to nosocomial infections among thousands of children in Romania, no country in the region was reporting many infections by 1994. This began to change with the first widespread outbreak of HIV in Ukraine and Belarus in 1995. The epidemic then started to take off in other countries of the region—Moldova in 1996 and the Russian Federation in 1998, followed by Latvia and then Kazakhstan. In the beginning of the 1990s, Russia had a low prevalence of HIV-infection. However, by the end of 1995, HIV began to spread rapidly in the Federation, reaching over 240,000 by mid-2003. Swift spread of HIV is now also evident in the Baltic countries (especially Estonia), Caucasus (Azerbaijan and Georgia) and Central Asia (Kazakhstan, Kyrgyz Republic, Tajikistan and Uzbekistan). While epidemiological and behavioral surveillance databases remain weak in many of the region's countries, there are increasing indications of a shift of the epidemic from highly vulnerable groups (such as needle-sharing IDUs and commercial sex workers) to the general population through sexual activity. In Ukraine, for example, where 75 percent of cumulative HIV infections are related to increasing drug use, the proportion of sexually-transmitted HIV infections is increasing. More people, mostly women, appear to be contracting HIV

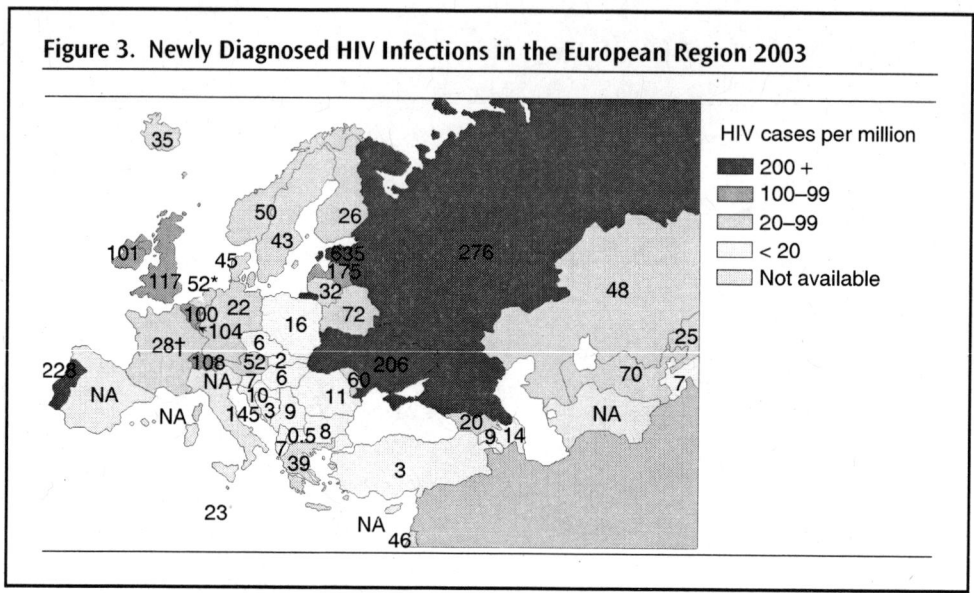

Figure 3. Newly Diagnosed HIV Infections in the European Region 2003

Source: EuroHIV 2003.

through sexual transmission and more pregnant women are testing positive for HIV, suggesting a shift of the epidemic into the wider population.

The Epidemiological Impact of HIV/AIDS Can be Significant

HIV/AIDS can have a significant epidemiological impact. The World Bank has conducted several studies of the potential impact of the epidemic in ECA countries (Lundberg 2001; Ruhel and others 2002; Godinho and others 2005). It is estimated that, in an optimistic scenario, mortality rates in Russia would increase from 500 per month to 21,000 per month in the period 2005–2020, and the cumulative number of HIV infected individuals would rise from 1.2 million to 5.4 million during the same period. In Central Asia, the initial slow growth of HIV, at monthly rates of 0.01–0.02, was followed in the late 1990s by a dramatic acceleration of the spread of HIV, with nearly a ten-fold increase in growth rates, primarily among injecting drug users. Research carried out in Kazakhstan, Kyrgyz Republic and Uzbekistan has revealed patterns of HIV growth strikingly similar to those observed in Russia, with the same potential epidemiological impact.

The HIV/AIDS Epidemic Can Reverse Economic Growth in the Region

Studies carried out by the Bank and other organizations suggest that an HIV epidemic is likely to have a far-reaching impact on the economic development of the region. With a generalized epidemic (prevalence over 1 percent), annual economic growth rates could decline by 0.5 to 1.0 percentage points. In addition, health expenditures could increase by 1-3 percent. A slow-down in GDP growth and losses in GDP level may be accompanied by losses in effective labor supply, which would be worsened by negative population growth in some countries. Table 2 shows the results of several modeling exercises carried out in the

---

Table 2. Modeling the Macroeconomic Implications of a Generalized AIDS Epidemic in the Russian Federation

The World Bank	▓ Dramatic impact in the absence of prevention/treatment
	▓ Mortality from 500/month in 2005 to 21,000/month in 2020
	▓ Cumulative HIV+ from 1.2 million in 2005 to 5.4 million in 2020
	▓ GDP falls 4.15% in 2010 and 10 in 2020
	▓ Prevention has a high cost-benefit as long as ARV price > $300/person/year
UNDP	▓ Significant population decline: 6.9 million (7%) loss by 2020
	▓ Population structure, dependency ratio distortion after 2010
	▓ Significant aggregate GDP declines (6%) over long term
	▓ Under open-economy, extractive industries more vulnerable
ILO	▓ **Scenario 1**: Epidemic remains constant: peak 685,000 HIV+ in 2007, 257,000 PLWA in 2012; disability and survivor pensioners grow 4–4.5% by 2010–2015
	▓ **Scenario 2**: Growing infection: peak 699,000 HIV+ in 2008, 259,000 PLWA in 2012, health care costs 0.26% GDP in 2011, disability benefits cost 7–8% in 2005–10
	▓ **Scenario 3**: Decreasing infection: peak 636,000 HIV+ in 2006, 255,000 PLWA in 2011, health care costs 0.25% GDP in 2011
	▓ **Scenario 4**: Infection probability shift: number of employed falls 0.1% 2005, 0.5% 2010 and 1.8% in 2050
	▓ **Scenario 5**: Complete risk group saturation: peak 1,169,000 HIV+in 2008, 181,000 PLWA in 2010, health care costs 0.43% GDP in 2011

Source: Sharp 2004.

Russian Federation. The Bank study in Russia estimated that, if decisive action were not taken to prevent a major epidemic, uninhibited spread of HIV would diminish the economy's long-term growth rate, taking off half a percentage point annually by 2010 and a full percentage point annually by 2020. As a consequence of decline in labor and capital inputs in Central Asia, GDP and GDP growth would be similarly affected. These studies also indicate that, at current prices, the costs of HIV treatment will not be sustainable by public budgets if the epidemic is not prevented, and/or treatment costs are not cut dramatically. As a policy implication, decisionmakers are advised to launch prevention programs, especially among highly vulnerable groups.

Early Action to Control the HIV/AIDS Epidemic in ECA has been Slow

Despite the potential human and economic impact of even moderate epidemics, the ECA Region has been slow, in general, in taking early action to control the HIV/AIDS epidemic, for a variety of reasons: the low prevalence rates, high stigma associated with the most vulnerable groups, lack of knowledge about the epidemic and its potential consequences, competing priorities, and lack of resources and capacity. "Politicians, policymakers, community leaders and academics have all denied what was patently obvious—that the epidemic of HIV/AIDS would affect not only the health of individuals, but also the welfare and well-being of households, communities and in the end, entire societies" (Barnett and Whiteside 2002).

Two Options to Tackle HIV/AIDS

Countries that are faced with a potentially rapid spread of HIV/AIDS have two options:

- Implement comprehensive prevention and treatment programs early on while prevalence rates are still low (Bonnel 2000); or
- Delay adopting and implementing evidence-based strategies and engaging on active prevention of HIV/AIDS until the epidemic becomes visible, with potentially serious impact on the health of the population and the economy.

If countries follow the first option, HIV/AIDS crisis could be averted through early and effective action, as it has happened in the European Union, United States, Australia, Brazil, Thailand, and Uganda. However, if countries opt for the second approach, much of the development efforts supported by Governments, NGOs and bilateral and multilateral agencies could be jeopardized as a result of the health, social and economic burdens created by an unchecked HIV/AIDS epidemic.

Study Design

This study was carried out in the context of the South Eastern Europe Declaration on HIV/AIDS Prevention and the Millennium Development Goals (MDGs) on HIV/AIDS, which are relevant for the Balkans region as follows:

> To develop strategies that begin to address the factors that make individuals particularly vulnerable to HIV infection, including under-development, economic insecurity, poverty, lack of empowerment of women, lack of education, social exclusion, illiteracy, discrimination, lack of information and/or commodities for self-protection, and all types of sexual exploitation of women, girls and boys.

The present study was carried out in Albania, Bosnia and Herzegovina, Macedonia, Serbia and Montenegro, and Kosovo. The study assessed the need for further policy development and investments in early prevention of HIV/AIDS. It also reviewed the situation regarding sexually-transmitted infections, as other STIs facilitate the spread of HIV; and data on TB, as this is the main opportunistic infection of AIDS.

The study was carried out by reviewing existing statistics and literature on HIV/AIDS and STIs in the countries under study, and interviewing key stakeholders in the field. Statistics and reports from the Government, NGOs and international agencies working in the field were reviewed. Meetings with Government counterparts and international agencies representatives took place in each country. NGO roundtables were organized in the countries under study.

The quality of the study data varies, which limits the ability to draw inferences, especially in what concerns trends regarding HIV/AIDS and other STIs. The unreliability of official statistics is due to the inefficiency of the surveillance system. No reliable HIV sentinel and second-generation surveillance (seroprevalence and behavioral data) exists throughout the sub-region. UNICEF carried out a Rapid Assessment in 2001–2002 in South Eastern

---

Box 1: Study Objectives

▩ Identify priorities for early actions that should be undertaken in the Balkans to prevent the spread of HIV/AIDS, in the framework of the UN 'Three Ones': one national AIDS Strategy that drives alignment of all partners; one national AIDS authority to coordinate it, and one nationally-owned monitoring and evaluation system to serve the needs of all.

▩ Inform the Bank's policy dialogue and operational work to control HIV/AIDS in the Balkans; and

▩ Contribute to building up the regional partnership between Governments, civil society, UN agencies, and multilateral and bilateral agencies to prevent HIV/AIDS, sexually-transmitted infections, and TB, and to improve public health in this region.

Europe (Wong 2002a), which provided valuable information that is extensively quoted by this study. However, as the assessment was based on small samples, generalization is problematic. Despite this limitation, the study gives a reasonably clear picture of the challenges that the Western Balkans face to take early action to prevent and control an HIV/AIDS epidemic.

This paper provides an overview of HIV/AIDS and STIs in the Balkans, summarizing the study main findings and including main recommendations for further study and for early action to prevent an HIV/AIDS epidemic in the Balkans. The Profiles on HIV/AIDS in the Western Balkans include the following information for each country and territory under study: an epidemiological overview of HIV/AIDS and STIs; a review of contextual factors that increase the vulnerability to HIV/AIDS; and a review of Government and civil society action so far to prevent and control a potential epidemic.

CHAPTER 2

HIV/AIDS in the Western Balkans

Epidemiological Situation and Trends

Presently, these countries have an HIV/AIDS prevalence rate under 0.1 percent. The Balkans countries under study have reported about 2,000 HIV/AIDS cases since the beginning of the epidemic in 1985. In all countries, infection rates among males exceed that of females. The spread of the infection is mostly sexual, despite the concentration of the epidemic among injecting drug users (IDU) in Serbia. As in other countries in the region, the epidemic may evolve from this initial phase to a second phase of increased concentration among injecting drugs users, and then sexual transmission would become again the main route in a third, more generalized phase of the epidemic. Early active prevention at this stage would provide the best results.

However, these data have to be interpreted with caution. Unreliable data is a major problem in every country. Officially reported cases of infection and disease often represent only 10–20 percent of the real number of cases. This is attributable to the stigma associated with the disease and associated risk factors such as drug use, commercial sex work, and homosexuality; low level of awareness among highly vulnerable groups, health staff, and the general population about the epidemic and HIV prevention, which reduces voluntary testing; the low number of testing facilities especially outside capital cities; financial constraints to voluntary testing; legal prohibition of anonymous testing; ineffective institutional arrangements; and insufficient technical capacity in surveillance.

Due to the low number of cases, and unreliable statistics, it is difficult to predict epidemiological trends. However, in other regional countries with higher prevalence rates, such as Ukraine, Russia, Belarus, Moldova, and Kazakhstan, transmission was mainly sexual in the initial HIV cases identified; the situation changed in the mid-1990s, when the epidemic increased in this region, with the highest growth rates in the world, mostly among injecting

---

Box 2: The HIV/AIDS and STIs Situation in the Balkans Region

The incidence and prevalence of HIV/AIDS in the Balkans is very low, and it is difficult to identify clear patterns of transmission and possible trends. However, in Serbia there is a concentration of the epidemic among injecting drug users (IDU); and in Montenegro higher incidence has been reported among sailors and tourist workers. Other vulnerable groups include commercial sex workers, men who have sex with men, displaced people and, in some countries, international peacekeeping forces and workers. Youth in general is very vulnerable.

Despite the low incidence and prevalence, the risk of an epidemic is quite significant. Underlying factors are in place that may fuel the epidemic by fostering an environment in which individuals are more likely to engage in high-risk behavior. The Balkans suffered severe conflicts that displaced thousands of people, brought international peacekeeping forces and international workers to the region, contributed to increased poverty and unemployment, especially among young people, and facilitated trafficking of women and children and commercial sex work. Levels of knowledge about the epidemic and prevention of HIV/AIDS are very low. In addition, war conflicts and the transition to a market economy have contributed to the decay of public health services and delayed the establishment of appropriate networks for HIV prevention.

---

drug users. This was due to the pervasive practices of sharing infected needles and syringes, and using infected blood in the preparation of the drugs for injection. Since 2000, however, the proportion of IDUs among HIV cases has been decreasing, while the proportion of cases due to sexual transmission has been increasing. This suggests that the epidemic has begun to spread to the general population through sexual contact—as it is already being observed in Serbia.

In Albania, over 70 percent of notified cases are thought to have acquired the infection abroad, which highlights the impact of migration. However, prevalence of hepatitis B (65 percent) and C (18 percent) antibodies among tested drug users is the highest in the region, indicating that sharing needles is a common practice. Analysis of the short-term trend shows an increase in the number of women registered with HIV and leveling off among men. This suggests both the potential for an epidemic of HIV among IDU, concomitantly with sexual transmission.

Box 3: Epidemiological Trends

In the Balkans, a potential epidemic may develop in one of three ways:

- Following the pattern of the epidemic in other regional countries, it becomes clearly concentrated on IDUs in the near future, until eventually it spreads to other groups of the population through sexual contact;

- Injecting drug use does not become widespread, and sexual transmission continues to be the most likely route of transmission of the infection and establishment of the epidemic; or

- An epidemic is prevented through early concerted efforts of public sector, NGOs, and the international community in close cooperation with young people at high risk of being infected or that are already infected. In this scenario, highly vulnerable groups reduce the harm of injecting drugs by avoiding associated risky practices such as sharing needles and syringes; and both highly vulnerable groups and vulnerable groups such as youth increase their knowledge about the epidemic and adopt safe sex practices.

The adult HIV prevalence in Bosnia and Herzegovina is still under 0.1 percent. However, authorities fear that the registered cases may only represent the "tip of the iceberg," primarily due to insufficient surveillance of risk groups, and that they will be able to detect the epidemic only at the point when it has fully developed and is hard to manage.

Macedonia also has an official low prevalence of HIVAIDS, and the transmission route for most of the registered cases is sexual. However, registered drug users are about 5,000– 6,000, and it is estimated that the country has about 20,000 drug users, of which 15,000 would be IDUs, which poses the risk of concentration of the epidemic among IDU in the near future.

Available data suggest that HIV prevalence in Serbia is low. However, these figures grossly underestimate the actual number of HIV infections due to insufficient surveillance data. Surveys indicate that IDU account for about half of the infections, although the proportion of these cases has been slightly decreasing, which usually suggests that the epidemic outbreak is spreading to other groups of the population through sexual transmission.

About 14 percent of all 55 officially registered cases in Montenegro occurred among tourist workers and another 14 percent among sailors. Geographically, one-third of all cases are from Podgorica, which is the most densely populated area in Montenegro, and almost one-half from costal municipalities, which is the area mostly visited by tourists. Injecting drug use seems to be less widespread than in Serbia. Therefore, in Montenegro, prevention of sexual transmission seems to be the most important priority.

No reliable data are available for the UN-administered territory of Kosovo. Little is known about the true prevalence of HIV/AIDS, and discerning trends in HIV/AIDS in Kosovo is essentially impossible, given the lack of HIV surveillance data and inherent flaws in AIDS case reporting.

All Balkans countries report much lower levels of sexually-transmitted infections (syphilis and gonococci infections) than the EU average (which is 1.5 per 100,000 population for syphilis). This is mainly attributable to the poorly developed surveillance and diagnostic systems, as well as lower accessibility and affordability of health services in the countries included in the study.

Tuberculosis is the main opportunistic infection for AIDS. TB case notification rates in the Balkans vary from 18 per 100,000 in Albania to 63 per 100,000 in Bosnia-Herzegovina. Again, this reflects more the weaknesses in the public health systems of these countries, especially on surveillance, than the real situation. Most countries report that the WHO-recommended approach DOTS has been adopted, but it is unclear what is the extent of implementation of this approach.

Vulnerable Groups

In the last five years, UNICEF and other international organizations carried out several surveys of knowledge, attitudes and practices (KAP) regarding HIV/AIDS. In 2001–2002, UNICEF carried out a Rapid Assessment and Response (RAR) on HIV/AIDS Among Especially Vulnerable Young People in Albania, Bosnia and Herzegovina, Croatia, and Serbia and Montenegro (Wong 2002a). This is the most important HIV/AIDS KAP study carried out so far in the region, and this study refers to it extensively. However, the scope of

---

Box 4: Vulnerable Groups and Their Awareness Regarding HIV/AIDS and STIs

There is considerable evidence of high levels of risk behavior among young people in the Balkans (see Table 68 on Vulnerable Groups). Levels of knowledge about HIV/AIDS and other STIs among the population appear to be low, especially among injecting drug users, commercial sex workers, men who have sex with men, prisoners, sailors, tourist workers, seasonal workers and other migrants, trafficked people, refugees and displaced people. In addition, there are high levels of stigmatization and medicalization of HIV and STI in the region. The present study has revealed an acute need for behavioral and serological surveillance of groups at increased risk of infection. This data would assist identifying priorities for designing preventive interventions for HIV/AIDS in the Balkans.

UNICEF's RAR is limited to some highly vulnerable groups, and the number of people surveyed in each group may not be sufficient to allow generalizing the findings to wider populations within each group. It would be important to pursue this work with larger samples, to have a better picture of the risk situation in the Balkans. DFID is now financing improvements in behavioral and serological surveillance among groups at risk, especially injecting drug users, in Serbia and Montenegro; CDC is also providing assistance to improvements in surveillance in some of these countries. Therefore, more complete information may become available in the near future.

In Albania, transmission is mostly sexual among the few registered HIV/AIDS cases. However, UNAIDS estimates that Albania has about 30,000 drug users, of which 70 percent would be IDUs, which could trigger a concentrated epidemic among this group. Although about a third of the population in Albania considered in a survey that HIV/AIDS is an important issue, KAP surveys carried out in the country have identified low level of knowledge and low level of condom use, especially among groups at risk, which could fuel a potential epidemic. For example, 47 percent of IDUs refer having between 2–5 sex partners per year; and 62 percent of CSW refer having between 50–100 sex partners per year. However, only 33 percent of men report ever having used condoms, and only 12 percent of CSW report always using condoms.

In 2003, the Bank carried out in Albania a qualititative poll of selected opinion leaders and a quantitative survey of 1,000 people nationwide, aged 15–59, to check the level of awareness and attitudes regarding HIV/AIDS in the country. The main results of this study, which are presented in the box below, show that Albanians are highly aware of HIV/AIDS but know little about the disease and its potential impact (Felzer 2004).

The UNICEF RAR indicated that youth in Bosnia and Herzegovina is at high risk of HIV/AIDS, especially injecting drug users and men who have sex with men. About 37 percent of IDUs were positive for Hepatitis C, which indicates sharing of needles, and about 70 percent reported sharing needles. However, 70 percent thought that they were not at risk of getting HIV/AIDS. In addition, stigma related with HIV/AIDS is widespread, which makes prevention activities difficult. In one survey, about 24 percent of women agreed with at least one of two discriminatory statements about people living with HIV/AIDS.

It is estimated that Macedonia has 12,000–15,000 IDUs, and that IDU overlap with CSW. High-risk behavior is reported among young people, IDUs, CSW, MSM and prisoners. More than half of injecting drug users report having 2–5 sexual partners. Among men who have sex with men, 30 percent report having 5–12 partners a year, and almost 60 percent report

---

Box 5: Public Opinion on HIV/AIDS in Albania

Opinion leaders and the general public

- Do not regard HIV/AIDS as requiring immediate attention;
- Welcome outside groups (international NGOs, multi/bi-laterals) to work on HIV/AIDS;
- Believe that improving the basic health infrastructure is of much more pressing importance than HIV/AIDS; and
- Are highly aware of the HIV/AIDS issue yet there are information gaps.

Opportunities and obstacles

- Growing openness in Albanian society provides an excellent opportunity to bring frank discussions in the public arena;
- But conservative and traditional attitudes are still prevalent;
- Resistance to condom use;
- Opinion leaders are very conscious of Albania's reputation while general public is more conscious about value of education;
- Great support for educational campaigns, especially in schools, however, no trust in school officials; and
- Crucial to pierce the sense of invulnerability that most people (including young people) have with regard to HIV/AIDS and to aggressively promote safe sex and condom usage.

Source: Felzer 2004.

never using a condom. About 40 percent of youth in general report having 2–5 sex partners per year, but the same percentage reports never or only sometimes using condoms.

It is estimated that Serbia has about 100,000 drug users, with 15 percent injecting drugs, of which more than half report sharing syringes and needles; and about one third report having sex with multiple partners, and never using condoms. In addition, there is overlap between IDUs, commercial sex workers and men who have sex with men. Among commercial sex workers, almost 60 percent report using drugs, and almost all report having had sex while on drugs. Among men who have sex with men, almost 80 percent report use of drugs. More than 60 percent of IDUs do not consider, however, drug use to be a risk factor. As in other countries, levels of knowledge are especially low among adolescents, and stigma associated with HIV/AIDS is high. The setting is conducive to a rapid increase in HIV infection.

In Montenegro, HIV cases were identified mostly among sailors and tourism workers, with the former group reporting high-risk sexual practices. About 1 percent of the Montenegro population are migrants. Injecting drug use is said to be low, but increasing drug use has been reported among children; the mean age of IDUs is 19 years; and almost 70 percent of IDUs report having 2–5 sex partners per year. In addition, 14 percent of commercial sex workers report injecting drugs. Low levels of knowledge about HIV/AIDS are reported among youth and health professionals. These factors potentially make the country vulnerable to HIV/AIDS and STI risk behaviors and epidemics.

Kosovo is estimated to have about 5,000 IDUs, who report high-risk practices conducive to the spread of the epidemic. Among youth 15–25 years, 80 percent knew that condoms and abstinence reduce the risk of HIV/AIDS, but only half of those having sex report using condoms always or most of the time, and mostly for preventing unwanted pregnancy.

The Context of Risk

The structural determinants to drive rapidly accelerating epidemics of STIs and HIV among young people are present in the Balkans. The extent and nature of risk practices and their structural determinants need urgently to be understood. The Balkans region is still unstable after a decade of armed conflicts; it is surrounded by countries where the HIV/AIDS epidemic is more advanced, such as Romania and Moldova; it has a high number of refugees and internally displaced persons (IDPs) in marginal conditions; and it is the pass-through of a significant amount of drug traffic to the rest of Europe, as well as human trafficking. The region is on the main drug traffic roads linking Asia and Western Europe, which enabled the growth of the IDU epidemic since 1995 in other regions in ECA. It is clear that injecting drug use in Eastern Europe has grown rapidly (tenfold) in the past decade (Soros 2002), and the potential for this risk behavior to fuel the HIV epidemic is enormous.

Human trafficking has become the third largest criminal business worldwide, after illegal drugs and weapons (Leimanowska 2002), and at least 175,000 women and girls were subject to this crime in ECA (including the Balkans) in 1997 alone. Increasing sexual commerce as a result of trafficking of women, high social stigmatization of sexual minorities and sex workers, which force them to operate underground, and the considerable number of refugees and IDUs living in poor sanitary conditions, without jobs, increase the risk of developing a rapid HIV/AIDS epidemic.

The Bank has recently carried out two studies that focus on youth and human trafficking in South East Europe (Cava and others 2004; Clert and others 2004) including countries that were assessed under this study. The first study shows that the quality of education is in general low, and unemployment is high among youth, while young people engage in risky practices such as consuming illegal drugs. The second study shows that young women, 18–24 years, from poor households in rural areas, with low educational level and precarious jobs are most at risk of being victims of trafficking. About 45 percent of identified cases of trafficking were from Albania. These two studies suggest that youth in the Balkans are at high risk of poverty, exclusion from social and formal labor networks, unemployment, trafficking—and therefore at high risk of becoming drug users, engaging in commercial sex work and becoming infected with HIV/AIDS and other STIs.

Box 6: Factors that Put Vulnerable Groups Most at Risk

The most striking feature in the Balkans is the high-risk environment. All major factors that could serve as contributing factors for the breakout of HIV/AIDS epidemic are present in the Balkans. Severe political instability, wars and consequent economic crisis and migration in this region over the last 10 years have generated poverty and presented overwhelming challenges which have affected all countries to varying degrees. These factors have also generated the structural conditions necessary to drive the very types of risk behavior and cultural shifts which create vulnerability to HIV and STIs, including: growth of injecting drug use; commercial sex work and migration; as well as breakdown of traditional family relationships and mores. At the same time, these countries have been making the transition from public health, education and welfare systems which were cast within the socialist mould; and endeavoring to reform these in the face of drastically reduced resource inputs to these systems.

Albania, Bosnia and Herzegovina, Macedonia, Serbia and Montenegro, and Kosovo have a population of about 20 million people. While all countries share the main epidemic drivers, there are also significant variations among them. Income per capita varies from less than $800 in Kosovo to almost $1,700 in Macedonia; unemployment varies from 15 percent in Albania to over 37 percent in Macedonia; people living under the poverty line range from 10 percent in Serbia and Montenegro to 50 percent in Kosovo.

In Albania, the population of the country grew from around 1.6 million in 1960 to 3.4 million in 2003. Albania is still one of the poorest countries in Europe, with GDP per capita around $1,400; one in four Albanians continues to live in poverty, despite strong economic growth over the past few years. This is a rural country (more than 50 percent live in rural areas), but undergoing rapid urbanization, which increases the risks for those moving from rural to urban areas. The population is young, and unemployment is high among youth, who account for half of poor people.

Recovering from the brutal war in the mid-1990s, Bosnia and Herzegovina has made significant strides in nation building and economic stability. However, the war caused widespread physical damage. Over 10 percent of the population was killed or wounded, and over half the population was displaced. Bosnia and Herzegovina has a mobile population due to migration,

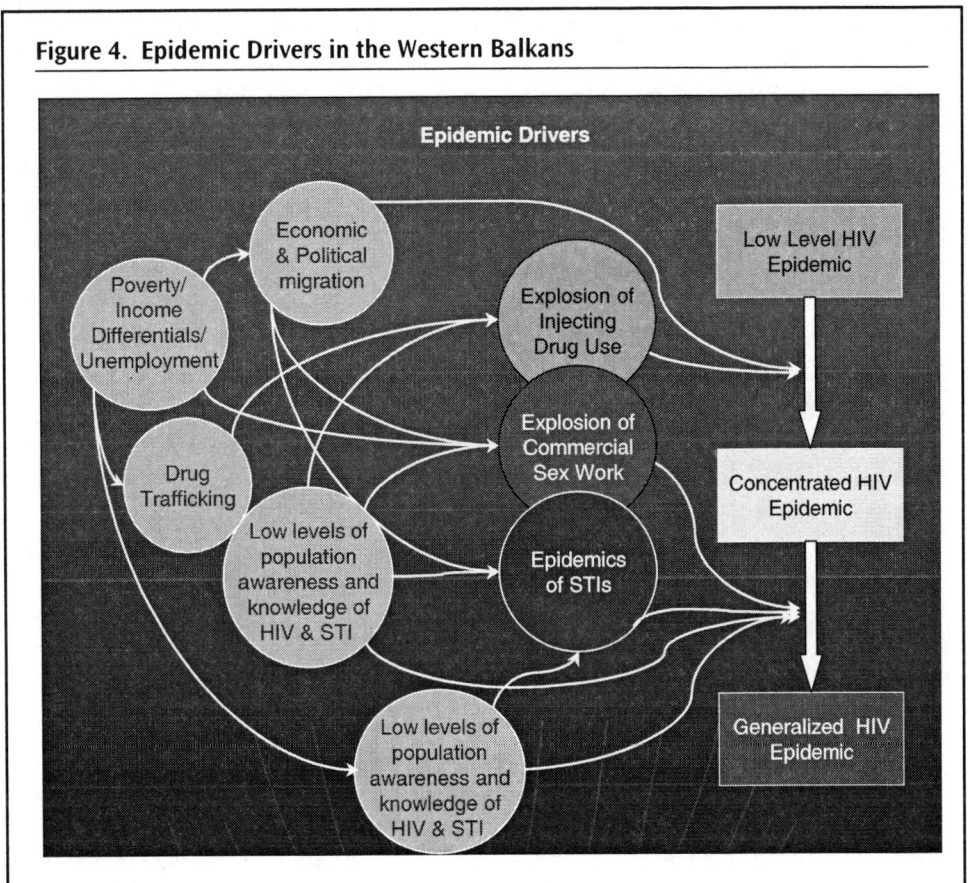

Figure 4. Epidemic Drivers in the Western Balkans

Source: Renton 2004.

including brain drain; 40 percent are unemployed, and uninsured; and 20 percent are living below the poverty level. Youth is especially affected by unemployment. In addition, Bosnia and Herzegovina had until recently a large presence of international troops.

The post-conflict environment of Macedonia has also created a favorable environment for HIV/AIDS and STIs epidemics. All risk factors are present, apparently more so than in other countries in this region, especially youth unemployment and women's trafficking from Moldova. Almost half of the unemployed are below 30 years of age. The country has 1,400 prisoners and more than 12,000 young men in the Army, as well as some foreign troops.

In Serbia and Montenegro, regional disparities and issues related with some vulnerable groups (ROMA, IDPs, refugees) put at risk achieving the Millennium Development Goals. Vulnerability to even small shocks remains high, putting vulnerable groups at risk of falling into absolute poverty. SAM gives priority to early accession to the EU, but face major obstacles.

Although Serbia has experienced a significant decrease in GDP, poverty is reported to affect 11 percent of the population, the lowest rate in the Balkans. Serbia has a young population—20 percent are below 15 years. As other countries in the region, Serbia is poised to experience a rapid increase in HIV/AIDS as a result of several factors: persistent post-conflict unemployment and increase in risk behavior, especially among young people; high population mobility; increased trafficking of drugs and humans, with low prevention and control; low knowledge about HIV/AIDS and risks; deterioration in health services and education; and lack of basic HIV/AIDS interventions. There is already a clear picture of a growing IDU epidemic, as well as a significant problem with commercial sex work and trafficking of humans—and overlapping of IDU and CSW.

In Montenegro, the general socio-economic status of the population has substantially declined over the last decade of political and economic instability, and economic transition. There has been a decrease in GDP, decreased production, increasing inflation and unemployment, and a growing informal economy. Women and youth may be at higher risk of poverty and unemployment than other groups. Although the country has avoided major conflicts, Montenegro became the residence for thousands of refugees from the former Yugoslav Republics and displaced people from Kosovo. Although many have returned to their original homes, the population structure and socio-economic conditions in Montenegro have changed.

Kosovo is a UN-administered territory. It has been reporting economic growth, which is partly due to migrant remittances and external aid. However, it remains one of the poorest regions in Europe, with 50 percent of the population considered poor and 12–15 percent considered extremely poor. Internal displacement of minority groups is a social problem, which aggravates poverty and leads to political instability. About half of the population—mostly young people—is not formally employed. Kosovo has a very young population; about 57 percent are below 25 years, which coupled with unemployment and other risk factors, significantly increases the risk of an HIV/AIDS epidemic. The weak economy, high migration, a large presence of international workers and troops, large numbers of internally displaced people (IDPs), returnees, commercial sex industry and trafficking are other risk factors. The region is said to be a transit site in the drug route from Afghanistan to Western Europe. Four years after the war, social and other services are returning to normal, but the events of the last decade have left this region vulnerable to HIV infection.

CHAPTER 3

National Responses to HIV/AIDS in the Western Balkans

Strategies and Regulatory Framework

Governments participated in the UN General Assembly Special Session (UNGASS) in June 2001; in the establishment of the Southeastern European (SEE) AIDS Initiative; and on the establishment of the Global Fund to Fight AIDS, Tuberculosis, and Malaria (GFATM). All Governments under the "The South Eastern Europe Declaration on HIV/AIDS Prevention" have agreed to take action to increase and prioritize national budgetary allocations for HIV/AIDS, and to ensure that existing resources and structures contribute optimally, and that all ministries and other relevant stakeholders make appropriate allocations (UNAIDS 2002a). This will include taking steps to integrate HIV/AIDS prevention, care, treatment, support and impact mitigation priorities into the mainstream of development planning, including poverty eradication strategies, gender equality strategies, national budget allocations, sector development plans and legislative reviews.

However, countries need to quickly act on these commitments to prevent the spread of the epidemic. Political leadership and decision-making capacity on HIV/AIDS are limited in the Western Balkans. Legislation is inadequate to support control efforts for preventing HIV spread, including on human rights and to overcome stigmatization of highly vulnerable groups. Therefore, the legal and regulatory framework, especially in relation to surveillance, prevention and control of HIV/AIDS and STIs need strengthening in all countries.

Albania has approved a Law on AIDS and established a National AIDS Committee. An AIDS Strategy has been approved, and the country has prepared a grant proposal to submit to the Global Fund. There is a pressing need to address and formulate strategic plans related to human and financial resources. In addition, an analysis of policies and procurement capacity regarding condoms, STI and TB drugs, antiretroviral drugs (ARVs), and HIV test kits is needed.

Box 7: Existing Strategies, Policies and Legislation

All Balkans countries have started taking action to prevent and control HIV/AIDS. However, early and appropriate action to prevent the HIV/AIDS and STIs epidemics varies from country to country. Most countries have prepared and approved HIV/AIDS Strategies, but have not financed adequately the respective Programs and Action Plans and have not received grants from the GFATM. Although Macedonia and Serbia have obtained grants from the GFATM, low political commitment and institutional capacity may hamper the use of available funds in these countries. Montenegro has not yet approved an AIDS Strategy, or obtained funding from the Global Fund.

Bosnia and Herzegovina's Parliament approved the AIDS Strategy in 2004, and is preparing to re-submit a proposal to the GFATM in 2005. A National AIDS Board has been established, and the UN-Theme Group is active in the country. A proposal for mandatory testing has been under discussion, as it raises human rights concerns.

In Macedonia, the completion of the national HIV/AIDS Strategy and the approval of the GFATM grant in 2003 represented a major breakthrough in strengthening the Government's response to HIV/AIDS. The process of application to the GFATM created incentives for establishment of the National Multisectoral HIV/AIDS Commission and the development of the national strategy. These processes also brought together the Government and NGOs addressing HIV/AIDS. However, the Republican Institute for Health Protection and the Clinic for Infectious Diseases, two key health institutions in Macedonia, have only recently been integrated into the overall planning process and implementation of the National AIDS Strategy. An AIDS Program has been developed, and the UN-Theme Group is active. The Government has initiated a review of the legal framework that is relevant for control of HIV/AIDS. Due to the political situation, however, political commitment to focus on HIVAIDS, STIs, and TB control in Macedonia is still low. Although the financial gap is less severe than in other regional countries in the short term, due to the GFATM grant, the weak institutional capacity to implement the grant and the National AIDS Program present significant risks for the prevention and control of a potential epidemic.

Serbia has already taken some crucial steps to address HIV/AIDS, including the establishment of the multi-sectoral Republican AIDS Commission and approval of a National Strategy in 2004, and it has successfully applied for GFATM funding. The UN-TG is very active in the country. The development of the National Policy Framework for HIV/AIDS and the GFATM grant proposal are key elements of the Serbia's strategy to combat the HIV/AIDS epidemic.

Montenegro has been preparing an AIDS Strategy, and has submitted a proposal for funding to the GFATM twice, but both times was advised to resubmit the proposal after revision. An AIDS Committee and an UN-Theme Group are active in Montenegro, as well as the public health network, but this territory clearly needs technical and financial assistance to finalize the Strategy and obtain a grant from the GFATM.

Kosovo has shown high commitment to control HIV/AIDS. A Strategy has been approved, involving various sectors and NGOs. Despite the civil conflict and then war through 1999, Kosovo established an AIDS Committee in December 2000 and developed an HIV/AIDS action plan in February 2004, but the plan has not yet been implemented because of lack of funding. Kosovo has reacted quickly to the recommendations of the UNICEF/WHO Rapid Assessment on substance abuse, establishing the Inter-ministerial Commission on Psychoactive Substances. A policy on illegal drugs is also under development. Moreover, the country recently adopted the Health Policy Guidelines for Kosovo, addressing five priorities for health care, among which is reducing communicable diseases, including HIV/AIDS. The country submitted a funding proposal for HIV/AIDS to the Global Fund, but was advised to resubmit a revised version.

Institutional Capacity to Tackle the Epidemic

The main issues regarding institutional capacity identified by the study are the following:

- Intervention projects with highly vulnerable groups (IDUs and CSW) and vulnerable groups (youth and migrants) are not well developed.
- The capacity to scale up existing successful harm reduction and other outreach programs (for example in Albania and Macedonia) is limited.
- Access to voluntary testing and counseling is very limited.
- Important public health functions, such as policy development, surveillance, and health promotion are not developed at all, or are weak.
- Services are fragmented and delivered *ad hoc* through all sections of the healthcare system including pharmacies.
- The burgeoning NGO movement refers limited funding, poor coordination, and lack of cooperation with the public sector.
- Laboratory infrastructure has declined; and well-validated diagnostics are not widely available.
- A significant proportion of young people are unemployed and uninsured, and therefore at higher risk of getting sick and not having access to care.

Box 8: Institutional Capacity to Prevent and Control these Diseases

Most Western Balkans countries have limited resources, underdeveloped, or dilapidated public health systems, and few NGOs to enable covering appropriately vulnerable groups and highly vulnerable groups. Institutional arrangements for public health are highly fragmented in most countries, an detached from policy and financing. This makes coordination and comprehensiveness very difficult within the health sector, let alone across sectors.

Although Macedonia and Serbia have obtained funding from the GFATM, and most other countries are preparing proposals to submit/re-submit to the Global Fund, implementation capacity is low throughout the Balkans countries. While Serbia has taken steps to manage the funds and implement the agreed work plan, Macedonia would require technical assistance to improve its implementation capacity. Education systems have not yet, in general, included sex education into the curricula.

Various NGOs in these countries provide activities in the areas where government support is lacking. However, local NGOs refer to lack of collective organization, and funding in some of the countries, and confirm that there is no cooperation among NGOs and the public sector for prevention of HIV/AIDS.

Regional conflicts have had a major impact on the development of surveillance systems. The reported incidence of HIV cases is believed to reflect only a small portion of all cases, and therefore prevalence estimates have lacked accuracy. Case notification systems have fallen into disuse, and there is consequently very little surveillance information which allows to understand trends of drug use, and HIV and STI incidence. However, it is crucial that the surveillance system is quickly upgraded to be able to report on risk behaviors, such as drug injecting and unsafe sex, and on real incidence and prevalence among vulnerable populations.

Voluntary testing and counseling is mostly absent in these countries and territories. Testing is not confidential and readily available at known locations, which drives patients to travel to other countries for testing (particularly to Serbia). In addition, the limited availability of treatment may also discourage vulnerable groups from being tested.

Although it is often stated that specialists do not use syndromic approaches to STI diagnosis and management, it is highly probable that management of diagnosis and management of STIs is largely syndromic given the restricted availability of diagnostic testing. However, the extent to which rational protocols are used to guide management is uncertain.

Treatment of people living with HIV/AIDS with antiretroviral drugs (ARV) is available in Albania, Macedonia and Serbia, but only for a few patients (less than 500). Costs of drugs and registration of drugs are high and prevent many countries except Serbia to import ARV drugs. However, there is a potential for cross-country registration to allow ARV drugs to be more easily imported and used. If the epidemic is not prevented, and the number of patients rises significantly in the near future, these countries will face the issue of financing treatment in addition to financing prevention.

In Albania, there are only four sentinel groups in Tirana, three testing sites, and one VCT site. No sex education has been included in school curricula, and treatment with antiretroviral drugs is available for only 50 patients. NGOs are very active in the country, but they are heavily dependent on external aid—a significant part of health funding comes from external sources. National HIV/AIDS planning is hampered by inadequate surveillance, inadequate information on HIV prevalence and dynamics, inadequate sexual and reproductive health education, and inadequate basic HIV/AIDS interventions. Control over common communicable diseases has been achieved to a certain degree in Albania, but sustained efforts are required to strengthen institutions to control the growing HIV/AIDS epidemic.

Bosnia and Herzegovina is now at the early stage of the efforts to combat HIV/AIDS. A recent assessment has found that a new reporting system implemented in 2003 in the Federation of Bosnia and Herzegovina should result in more complete case reporting and in collection of more relevant data (Archibald 2003). There is one methadone program in the country; and funding for ART therapy is being secured through Federal Solidarity funds in the Federation Bosnia and Herzegovina. The Bank-financed health projects have been supporting HIV/AIDS activities. Concurrently, numerous local NGOs have launched critical HIV/AIDS interventions directed at the most vulnerable groups in the country. However, there are few anonymous testing and VCT sites, and rates of testing are low. Finally, the ability of NGOs to sustain interventions is imperiled, as they depend heavily on external funding, which has been decreasing.

Macedonia is said to have a good surveillance system in place, but low reporting suggests otherwise. Blood is screened to ensure safe blood supply. Under the GFATM grant, the country plans to improve surveillance, and support the public system and the small, but active NGO network to work with youth and highly vulnerable groups; and the country aims at reaching 20 PLWHA with antiretroviral treatment within the next three years. Clinical guidelines and protocols of treatment, care and support for PLWHA have been prepared. However, the weak institutional capacity poses serious risk regarding the implementation of this grant.

In Serbia, many national institutions, NGOs and international agencies are supporting efforts to control the HIV/AIDS epidemic at this early stage. However, in Serbia testing rates are low; no youth-friendly services are in place; there is only one STI clinic in Belgrade; no methadone program has been established; sex education has not yet been included in school curricula; and only about 450 patients are on antiretroviral treatment. Several new programs, financed by the GFATM, and bilateral donors such as DFID and USAID, are supporting efforts to improve surveillance systems necessary to manage the HIV epidemic in Serbia, and to provide prevention services to youth and highly vulnerable groups. The results of a US Centers for Disease Control and Prevention (CDC) pilot study on surveillance within highly vulnerable populations should help health planners develop a functional HIV/AIDS surveillance system supported by rapid testing technologies that can be used for monitoring and evaluation of the epidemic. In addition, Serbia will participate in a new WHO-Euro Training Program in Second Generation Surveillance.

Montenegro faces both challenges and opportunities to establish institutional capacity for managing health sector and ensuring that essential public health functions are in place and well functioning, including protection from infectious diseases. Although HIV/AIDS testing is available in Montenegro, no sentinel and behavioral surveillance are yet in place. Prevention work with youth and harm reduction for IDUs are not yet available, and patients have to go to Serbia for treatment. Sex education has not been initiated in schools, but education on drug addiction has started. The small but active NGO sector has just started work with youth and highly vulnerable groups.

In addition to high commitment to prevent and control HIV/AIDS, Kosovo has been developing primary health care through a family medicine approach. However, access to services is still limited, as costs are high. Blood is screened, but testing of vulnerable and highly vulnerable groups is only available as part of training. There is no methadone program, and no treatment of opportunistic infections and HIV/AIDS. There is an STI clinic in Pristina, and sex education has just started. Many NGOs are present in the field, but there is still little work on HIV/AIDS. WHO has been supporting the development of sentinel and behavioral surveillance, and CIDA/Canada and USAID have also provided significant assistance, but donor support has been decreasing.

Resources for HIV/AIDS Prevention and Control

In general, in all countries funding available for prevention and treatment of HIV/AIDS, STIs and drug use, from public and private sources and from donors, only allows for limited research and pilot-based actions, and is inadequate to scale up activities to prevent a significant epidemic. In addition, donor coordination is very weak in the Western Balkans, making it hard to scale up from small, fragmented donor initiatives to comprehensive strategies. One of the countries in the grouping (Montenegro) has had major problems in

---

Box 9: Resources Available to Control these Diseases

Funding available from public budgets for prevention and treatment of HIV/AIDS and other STIs is limited in all countries with the exception in the short term of Macedonia and Serbia, as these countries have just received GFATM grants for the next two years.

International aid may be decreasing due to the end of the conflicts, and the need to provide support elsewhere (Africa, Afghanistan, Iraq). This seems to be the case with UNICEF and CIDA/Canada, which have been two major players on HIV/AIDS in the region. Serbia and Macedonia have already had successful applications to the GFATM, and all other countries have been preparing funding proposals to submit to the GFATM. DFID is providing significant support to Serbia and Montenegro.

However, even in the two countries that have obtained funding from the GFATM, the financial gap is still substantial, and weak institutional capacity to provide leadership and coordination of internal and external stakeholders, especially in health ministries, is a common feature in all countries.

---

mobilizing donor resources for health unlike other countries. All countries operate some type of social or publicly-funded health insurance scheme. In many of these countries, total spending on health is in general appropriate, but allocation of resources is inefficient and inequitable. In addition, private practice is increasing, with fees for service raising inequalities and driving costs of health care high. Details of public financing for HIV/AIDS activities is missing in most countries.

Albania has the lowest overall health expenditure as a percentage of GDP (2.6 percent in 2005), less than half the regional average, and lags behind other countries in the region and the European average of 4.8 percent. Public spending on health and education remains low by regional and international standards, and sector resources are not used effectively. In addition, a significant part of the health-funding still comes from external sources. Details of public funding for HIV/AIDS were not available.

Recorded public health expenditure on health in Bosnia and Herzegovina was 7.8 percent of GDP in 2003 and out of pocket expenditures amounted to 4.7 percent of GDP during the same year. The high expenditure on health is a reflection of the high cost of operating a fragmented, multi-tiered structure, the inefficient allocation of expenditures, clinically inefficient approach to care and a weak system of sector management. The international community continues to play an important role in Bosnia and Herzegovina, most notably through EUROFOR. Government expenditures remain dependent on international assistance and are increasingly unsustainable, with spending on new programs constrained by IMF and Bank limitations.

Public expenditure on health in Macedonia has ranged from 5.4 percent to 6.1 percent of GDP between 1999 and 2003, which is about the regional average. Although in the short term, Macedonia may have a lower resource gap for HIV/AIDS control than other countries in the region, due to the GFATM grant ($4.4 million for 2004–2006), issues of sustainability and implementation capacity are of concern, and Macedonia still faces an estimated resource gap of $4–$5 million.

In Serbia, public expenditure on health has been growing quite strongly in the last three years, and is projected to continue to grow at the rate of GDP. However, the increase

Table 3. Financing of Prevention and Treatment in the Western Balkans

Albania	Bosnia and Herzegovina	Macedonia	Serbia	Montenegro	Kosovo
Total health expenditure <3% of GDP	Total health expenditure 12.5% GDP	Public expenditure on health about 6% (1999–2003)	Total health expenditure 11% GDP	8% of budget is allocated to health	Public health expenditures 4.4 % GDP in 2003
Dependent on international assistance	Public expenditure on health 7.8% GDP	GFATM grant $4.4 million for 2004–2006	Public Health expenditure 6.1% GDP	25% out of pocket expenditure	The MOH provided funds for the Kosovo AIDS Office in 2002 and 2003, but the program is mostly donor-dependent
GFATM proposal not yet approved	Out-of-pocket costs 4.7% GDP	Estimated resource gap for HIV/AIDS of $4–$5 million	About $4 million for HIV/AIDS	MOH allocated about $350,000 for HIV in 2004	
	Dependent on international assistance		GFATM grant of $2.7 million	Estimated $2.5 million gap for 2005–2006	
	GFATM proposal not yet approved		DFID grant of $2.5 million		
				GFATM proposal not yet approved	GFATM proposal not yet approved

Source: Ministries of Finances and Health Insurance Funds 2003.

has not kept pace with health expenditures, with the Health Insurance Fund facing chronic financial stress and accumulated arrears totaling about 1 percent of GDP. On HIV/ AIDS, the Government allocates about $4 million for blood testing, and treatment of about 300 HIV/AIDS patients (at $10,000–$12,000/patient). Serbia has been awarded a GFATM grant of $2.7 million, and a DFID grant of $2.5 million for HIV/AIDS. EAR and OSI are providing assistance to the establishment of a School of Public Health. UNAIDS, UNICEF, USAID/CDC and CIDA/Canada have been providing active assistance on prevention of HIV/AIDS.

Montenegro allocates about 8 percent of its budget to health. A UNDP survey estimated that 25 percent of health expenditures were out of pocket. The MOH allocated about $350,000 in 2004 for communicable diseases to HIV testing and other prevention activities. Montenegro is now preparing a revised proposal for the GFATM to support public health activities to control HIV and TB infections with specific emphasis on high-risk groups; and to co-finance part of the estimated $2.5 million needed for two years. Although donor support has been limited, the territory is expected to benefit from the $2.5 million DFID grant for work with vulnerable groups in Serbia and Montenegro.

Public health expenditures in Kosovo are relatively low. According to Government estimates, in 2003, public health expenditures were 4.4 percent of GDP, which is below the regional average and well below neighboring countries with the exception of Albania. Prospects for 2003–2005 are for a very small increase of public expenditure in absolute terms (less than 5 percent in three years). The MOH provided some funding for the Kosovo AIDS Office in 2002 and 2003, but the program is mostly donor-dependent.

International Support

Several organizations have been providing financial and/or technical assistance for research and interventions to control HIV/AIDS and STIs in the region: UN agencies, bilateral agencies such as USAID, CIDA (Canada) and DFID (UK), and international NGOs such as the Soros Foundation/OSI and Project Hope. However, international support varies from country to country, and does not cover all key areas. Donor coordination is weak, and many donors are leaving this region as demand from other regions (Africa, Afghanistan, Iraq) has been increasing recently.

UNAIDS has supported the establishment of UN-Theme Groups (UN-TGs) in all countries; and has provided support to the development of HIV/AIDS Strategies, and country-applications for grants from the Global Fund Against AIDS, TB and Malaria. However, UNAIDS faces difficulties, for example in Serbia, to finance activities agreed by the UN-TG.

UNICEF was one of the most active agencies in the Western Balkans, providing support to youth in general through schools and NGOs. However, it is scaling down its operations in this sub-region as it faces increased demand from other regions. UNICEF carried out the Rapid Assessment of knowledge, attitudes and practices among groups at risk in South Eastern Europe, which although based on small samples, provided initial valuable information about the epidemic and risk practices in the Western Balkans.

WHO has been supporting capacity building for surveillance, and for updating treatment protocols.

Under the Regional Strengthening of Essential Public Health Functions in the Balkans project, CIDA/Canada financed and the Canadian Public Health Association provided technical assistance in the Western Balkans to: (i) strengthen HIV/AIDS and STI surveillance systems, including rapid assessments of the surveillance system, and technical advice and training in surveillance methods and data analysis and interpretation; (ii) support skills building in health promotion strategies and best practices related to voluntary counseling and testing, HIV prevention, and AIDS care and support; and (iii) mapping of care, support, and treatment process for PLWHA.

DFID has been focusing on EU-association policies and processes, and aid effectiveness. On HIV/AIDS, the agency has been financing work with highly vulnerable groups in Serbia and Montenegro, with a planned allocation of $2.6 million over two years. The HIV Prevention among Vulnerable Populations Initiative (HPVPI) in Serbia and Montenegro started in 2004. Implementing partners for this Initiative are the Open Society Institute (New York), the Imperial College (London, UK), and the UNDP Belgrade Office. However, DFID aims to graduate from programs in the Western Balkans between 2007–2010.

USAID has been supporting a cross-border project in Bosnia and Herzegovina, Macedonia, Romania, Croatia, and Bulgaria. Through RiskNet, Population Services International (PSI) supports NGOs engaging in prevention activities, including referrals to treatment centers; VCT; and distribution of condoms, clean needles (not funded by USAID), and educational materials. USAID has also financed CDC activities in Serbia to improve surveillance of HIV/AIDS and other communicable diseases. As other agencies, USAID has been scaling down its support in the Western Balkans.

International NGOs have been supporting the growing NGO sector engaged in prevention activities with vulnerable and highly vulnerable groups, and providing support to the self-help movement among drug users and people living with HIV/AIDS, but lack the financial and human capacity to scale up these activities throughout the region.

The Soros Foundation/OSI has been active in the sub-region, supporting the first harm reduction programs in the Western Balkans. These efforts have been successful in Albania and Macedonia, and OSI is now providing support to the development of similar programs in Serbia and Montenegro, as mentioned above. Another NGO that has been providing support in the Western Balkans, with financing from SIDA/Sweden for 2004–2007, is Project Hope. Project Hope is making available reliable and verifiable data; and improving the NGO and public services capacity to respond to the epidemic. The first training workshop was organized in Zagreb in 2004.

The Bank has now started to provide some assistance to this group of countries to prevent HIV/AIDS. HIV/AIDS control is included in the Poverty Reduction Support Credit in Albania, which is providing assistance to the development of strategic planning. In Bosnia and Herzegovina, the Bank-financed Basic Health Project financed HIV/AIDS prevention activities and the new project—Health Scale Up Project will also support HIV/AIDS-related activities. In Kosovo, a Youth Grant will include youth friendly centers that will engage on prevention of HIV/AIDS. The chapter on the Bank role makes recommendations for scaling up Bank support for prevention of HIV/AIDS in the Western Balkans.

CHAPTER 4

Recommendations for Region-Wide Activities

Decreasing the risk of an HIV/AIDS epidemic spreading throughout the Balkans region, and becoming a long-term development problem as it has happened in other regions, requires a mix of interventions aimed at reducing the risk of infection in the short term, and interventions aimed at tackling structural factors in the medium to longer term. Activities in the short term would aim at ensuring the adoption of evidence-based, cost-effective strategies for prevention of HIV/AIDS; improving the quantity, quality and use of the information available; and scaling up coverage of the most vulnerable groups with harm reduction and safe sex programs. The sustainability of these actions requires improvement of public health services in the medium term. Longer-term interventions would aim at preventing poverty, exclusion and unemployment, for example, by empowering young people to participate in the regional and global labor market.

The table below identifies four key priority areas of action to reduce risks of a generalized epidemic in the region. These include (i) establishment of a political and social environment favorable to prevention and control of HIV/AIDS, especially among the most vulnerable groups; (ii) making essential information about the epidemic available and used in decision-making about prevention and control; (iii) carrying out cost-effective prevention activities; and (iv) providing sustainable care and social support of good quality to people living with HIV/AIDS.

Actions for the short, medium, and long term are indicated below. Most of the recommendations are addressed to Governments, although some are also addressed to NGOs and international organizations (as indicated).

> **Box 10: Main Gaps Identified by the Study**
>
> - The majority of the Balkans countries have approved AIDS Strategies, but most Governments have limited political will, leadership and technical capacity and/or funding to implement them.
> - Most Governments have not made any specific allocation for HIV/AIDS prevention.
> - Only Macedonia and Serbia have obtained grants from the GFATM, while other international aid has been decreasing.
> - Information about the most vulnerable groups, including data about knowledge and practices, is scant. Routine surveillance does not provide appropriate data, and behavioral and sentinel surveillance of HIV/AIDS and STIs have not yet been established.
> - Knowledge about the epidemic is very low among most vulnerable groups and general population.
> - Practices reported by the most vulnerable groups involve a high risk of infection.
> - Epidemic drivers such as trafficking of women and drugs, drug use and commercial sex work put youth at increased risk.
> - Public health services in these countries are under-funded and have low capacity, and therefore do not fulfill key public health functions such as policy development, surveillance and prevention including of HIV/AIDS.
> - The most vulnerable groups (IDUs, CSWs and others) have not been covered, or have only been covered by pilot projects. For example, although there is higher incidence of HIV/AIDS among sailors and tourist workers in Montenegro, prevention activities targeted at these groups have not been developed.
> - Countries that have allocated funding for treatment are only able to cover a small number of patients.

Actions for the Short Term

Implementation of HIV/AIDS Strategies

The Western Balkans countries have approved HIV/AIDS Strategies (with the exception of Montenegro), and have agreed to establish national prevention targets as part of the national planning process. The specific recommendations in this area are:

- Implement approved AIDS Strategies in Albania, Bosnia and Herzegovina, Kosovo, Macedonia and Serbia; and approve an evidence-based, cost effective Strategy in Montenegro.
- UNAIDS, Bank and other partner organizations may want to consider providing technical assistance to Montenegro to finalize the preparation of the HIV/AIDS Strategy.
- Support legislative and policy development to:
  - Facilitate the work with highly vulnerable groups such as IDUs, MSM, CSW, and other vulnerable populations. For example, anonymous testing should be legalized in Montenegro.
  - Promote prevention, treatment and reporting of HIV/AIDS and STI cases.

Leadership and Decision Making

Periodic policy review, as well as review of surveillance and program evaluation data are necessary to provide continuous quality improvement as HIV/AIDS prevention and control

Table 4. Four Key Priority Areas for Action

Decreasing risks of HIV/AIDS	Highly vulnerable groups[5]	Young people in general
Favorable political and social environment	▩ Human rights and anti-discrimination laws ▩ Harm reduction and safe sex policies ▩ Decriminalization of drug use	▩ Human rights ▩ Anti-trafficking of humans and drugs ▩ Information ▩ Safe sex policies ▩ Education and training ▩ Employment ▩ Poverty alleviation
Essential information	▩ Behavioral surveillance: needle-sharing and unsafe sex	▩ Behavioral surveillance ▩ KAP and unsafe sex
Prevention of HIV	▩ Information ▩ Youth Centers ▩ School-based education ▩ VCT ▩ Peer-to-Peer-education about drug use and STIs ▩ Safe sex programs including condom social marketing ▩ Drug replacement therapy ▩ Harm reduction programs	▩ Information ▩ Youth Centers ▩ School-based education ▩ VCT ▩ Peer-to-Peer-education about drug use and STIs ▩ Safe sex programs including condom social marketing
Sustainable care and social support of good quality	▩ STI treatment ▩ Prevention of MTCT ▩ Appropriate care & social support for PLWHA	▩ STI treatment ▩ Prevention of MTCT ▩ Appropriate care and social support for PLWHA

programs are implemented. Without incorporation of surveillance and evaluation data on a continuous basis, public health and treatment programs will not adequately address existing highly vulnerable groups nor respond to changes in the epidemic as it passes from the highest risk groups to the general population.

▩ Training for policymakers and health leaders should include leadership development, and skill building to use data for decision making.
▩ International organizations may want to consider co-financing this training. WHO and other partner organizations have been providing training in surveillance in Zagreb. The World Bank Institute provides training in leadership and decision-making.

---

5. Highly vulnerable groups include injecting drug users, commercial sex workers, trafficked people, men who have sex with men and prisoners. Other vulnerable groups include migrants, soldiers and peacekeeping forces and other mobile populations.

Box 11: Main Priorities for Early Action

Actions for the Short Term

- Implementation of approved HIV/AIDS Strategies.
- Adoption of sound policies for treatment of people living with HIV/AIDS.
- Fund-raising and allocation of budgetary funds for HIV/AIDS prevention.
- Establishment of behavioral and sentinel surveillance throughout the region.
- Information and education of young people, especially most vulnerable groups.
- Scaling up coverage of most vulnerable groups such as injecting drug users, commercial sex workers, men who have sex with men, sailors, tourist and seasonal workers, and migrants with harm reduction and safe sex programs

Actions for the Medium Term

- Investments on public health services to enable them to perform key public health functions such as policy development, surveillance and prevention including of HIV/AIDS; which ensure the sustainability of actions taken in the shorter term.
- Improvement of opportunities for young people that decrease risks associated with epidemic drivers such as unemployment, trafficking of people and drugs, use of drugs and commercial sex work; and enable young people to participate in the regional and global knowledge economy.

Fund-raising and Allocation of Budgetary Funds for HIV/AIDS Prevention

Financial gaps were identified by this Study even in countries that are benefiting from GFATM grants. On the other hand, increased costs of prevention and treatment will not be sustainable in any of these countries, but especially in poorer regions such as Montenegro and Kosovo. Therefore, Governments are advised to rise funding for HIV/AIDS that would allow them to sustain some of the necessary key actions.

- Albania, Bosnia and Herzegovina, Montenegro, and Kosovo should re-submit proposals for funding to the Global Fund Against AIDS, TB and Malaria and other sources of funding.
- UNAIDS, the Bank and other partner organizations may want to consider financing technical assistance to prepare these grant proposals.
- Inter-sectoral committees on HIV/AIDS should be involved in decision making of Government resource allocation and monitoring of flow of funds.
- Increase public funding and resources available for HIV/AIDS prevention and treatment to contain the spread of the epidemic.
- Provide financial incentives and better reimbursement rates for the provision of public health services to displaced people, particularly for anonymous testing and counseling.
- Improve financial planning and resource transfer mechanisms from Governments to NGOs and the private sector for provision of HIV/AIDS related services.

Establishment of Behavioral and Sentinel Surveillance Throughout the Region

UNICEF, CIDA/Canada, DFID and USAID, through CDC, have been providing some support to the development of second-generation surveillance (seroprevalence and behavioral surveillance) and sentinel surveillance in the region. However, this is a typical public responsibility that should constitute a high priority for the regional Governments in terms of budgetary allocation, fund-raising and capacity building. Two key recommendations are indicated below.

- Start regional cooperation on reporting HIV/AIDS and STI cases back to the country of residence anonymously. The anonymous form would include information on sex and age, and sub-region of residence in the home country and risk group/route of transmission.
- Develop second-generation surveillance, including behavioral surveillance, among groups at risk, such as CSWs, IDUs and prisoners; and antenatal clinic and family planning attendees.
- EuroHIV, which reports on data from all Western Balkans countries, would be able to provide technical assistance to improve regional surveillance; and the European Union may want to consider co-financing this activity as these countries are in the EU neighborhood.

Information and Education of Young People, Especially Most Vulnerable Groups

In most countries in the region, the main route of transmission is sexual; the most vulnerable groups, youth and the general population reveal a low level of knowledge about the epidemic and prevention in general; and youth is very vulnerable to epidemic drivers. Civil societies (through NGOs), Governments and agencies assisting them should therefore increase the efforts to inform and educate them. Some of the areas in which action should be taken are indicated below.

- Support a comprehensive program of information and education about HIV/AIDS and STIs in partnership with NGOs, especially among vulnerable and highly vulnerable groups, and through the education system.

Box 12: MDG Indicators Relevant for the Western Balkans

Target 7: Have halted by 2015 and begun to reverse the spread of HIV/AIDS

1. Condom use at last high-risk sex;
2. Percentage of population aged 15–24 years with comprehensive correct knowledge of HIV/AIDS; and
3. Contraceptive prevalence rate.

- Increase access of young people to youth-friendly services that will provide infor-
mation and education about HIV/AIDS and other sexually-transmitted infections
(STIs); and to commodities such as condoms and syringes and needles.
- Increase availability of affordable, and confidential/anonymous testing services
through partnership of the public system with private providers.
- Provide training and support in client-focused confidential STI and HIV service
provision.
- Provide testing and treatment of STIs and HIV/AIDS outside capital cities.
- UNICEF and the AIDS Foundation East West (APHEW) may consider providing
technical assistance in the above-mentioned areas. APHEW has developed a train-
ing program on voluntary testing and counseling, which has been provided in
Ukraine and Moldova.

Scaling Up Coverage of Most Vulnerable Groups

It is urgent to expand HIV prevention among vulnerable groups such as injecting drug
users, sex workers, men who have sex with men, sailors, tourist and seasonal workers, and
migrants, especially through harm reduction and safe sex programs, in order to prevent
the transmission of HIV. While Serbia and Macedonia have funding from GFATM, and
Serbia is benefiting from a DFID grant for work with injecting drug users, other countries
do not have the ability to scale up these key programs unless they equally obtain grants.
Therefore, fund-raising takes priority to enable expanding work with the most vulnerable
groups, which should include expanding access to information, condoms, life skills education, voluntary counseling and testing, access to clean needles, substitution therapy and
other youth-friendly services. Key actions are listed below:

- Scale up outreach programs targeted at vulnerable and highly vulnerable groups
through partnerships of the public system, NGOs, and international organizations.
- Train former drug users and commercial sex workers to engage in peer education
about harm reduction and safe sex.
- Provide services for pregnant women to prevent mother-to-child transmission of
HIV/AIDS.
- The Soros Foundation/OSI is the most experienced organization in the region on
outreach programs, especially harm reduction programs. Public services and NGOs
that want to engage on, or scale up, these activities should consider visiting successful programs in Albania, Macedonia and Serbia that have been supported by OSI.
- Donors may want to consider financing the scaling up of successful outreach
programs, such as harm reduction programs, which are one of the most effective
activities to prevent an epidemic.

Develop Policy on Treatment of HIV/AIDS Cases with Antiretroviral Drugs

While the poorest Western Balkans countries and territories are not able to provide
publicly-financed treatment even of opportunistic infections, some (Albania, Macedonia,
Serbia) have started providing treatment of HIV/AIDS with antiretroviral drugs at a cost
of about $10,000 per patient per year. However, while demand for treatment will increase

in the future, entirely financing it from the public budget will not be sustainable if the number of cases increases significantly. Governments may want to consider the following actions:

- Adopt evidence-based policies on antiretroviral treatment recommended by WHO and UNAIDS, to ensure equity and prevent misuse of these drugs that may cause drug resistance.
- Improve procurement planning for antiretroviral drugs, introduce tender procedures for the provision of ARV drugs and negotiate prices of ARV drugs with manufacturers to reduce the overall spending on drugs and consumables and free resources for additional prevention and treatment.
- Open provision of pharmaceuticals to the private sector.

Actions for the Medium and Long Term

Investments on Public Health Services

Considerable investment is needed in the public health systems in these countries to enable them to perform key functions such as policy development, surveillance and prevention; and to ensure the sustainability of actions taken in the shorter term to avoid a major HIV/AIDS epidemic. In the six countries and territories under study, strengthening capacity and developing sound institutions in the public and NGO sectors is essential, and will require a concerted and long-term effort to reduce fragmentation of institutional responsibility and donor effort, and to modernize leadership and management so as to unleash the potential of a sizable and young public health workforce. Many partner organizations have been involved in capacity building in key public health functions in this sub-region, including by developing the School of Public Health in Serbia; the Andrija Stampar School of Public Health, in Zagreb, WHO, USAID/CDC, CPHA, and Soros. In addition, the EU has a strong public health program and has started making investments in this area in Serbia. Key recommendations for Governments and agencies that provide assistance to them are indicated below.

- Build technical capacity in the public health system, especially in Institutes of Public Health in each country and territory.
- Modernize leadership and management of public health services.
- Support training activities for staff from public health services and NGOs at the Andrija Stampar School of Public Health.
- Support the development of the School of Public Health in Serbia.
- The EU may want to consider co-financing efforts to improve public health in the Western Balkans.

Improve Opportunities for Young People

Economic reform and improvement of living standards are crucial yet highly vulnerable to external shocks. These countries are facing numerous, competing priorities, and doing so in a highly unstable region. However, longer-term strategies should focus on decreasing risks associated with unemployment among young people, trafficking of people and drugs, use of drugs and commercial sex work; and which enable young people to participate in the regional and global labor markets. Many national and international agencies work in these areas, including among others UNICEF, UNFPA, UNODC, and IOM. The Bank has prepared a Note on mainstreaming youth issues in ECA that provides detailed recommendations in this area; it has been considering financing youth operations, which would include activities aimed at (i) improving inclusion and empowerment; (ii) risk reduction; and (ii) income-generation; and many of its activities in the Western Balkans will have an impact on living standards of young people (Cava and others 2005; and see Chapter 5). The EU may also be able to have an increased role in this area.

Specific Actions for Countries and Territories

Recommendations for priority actions for early prevention of HIV/AIDS in each country or territory under the Study are presented below. The most urgent actions are highlighted in Table 1. The majority of the proposed actions are similar in all countries, with a few variations according to the specific situation in each country.

Albania. Albania should fund and implement the National HIV/AIDS Strategy that has been recently approved. In Albania, the transport and mining sectors are growing. Country projects in these areas could coordinate with the health sector and other stakeholders to raise awareness, conduct peer education, and expand condom distribution for truckers, CSWs, and bar/hotel owners. The Government should explore mechanisms to work effectively with civil society groups (NGOs working with most vulnerable groups, private industry including transport and mining). The basic public health infrastructure should be improved in Albania. This includes surveillance systems, information and education activities, training of health professionals in VCT, drug abuse treatment, and treatment of opportunistic infections. In addition, guidelines for voluntary testing and counseling, prevention of mother-to-child transmission, and treatment of people living with HIV/AIDS and for STIs should be updated according to WHO/UNAIDS recommendations.

Bosnia and Herzegovina. Critical next steps include implementing and financing the broad HIV/AIDS Strategy prepared by the National AIDS Board. This must be done in close collaboration with civil society, underscoring the vital need for high-quality and timely HIV surveillance data, especially second-generation surveillance data. Genuine integration of HIV/AIDS into national (and administrative entity) planning mechanisms is also critical. Undertaking these tasks in the context of Bosnia and Herzegovina's administrative complexity and weak governance will be a major challenge. However, as the country struggles to refine its service delivery sectors, including public health, there is an opportunity to ensure that HIV/AIDS will be thoughtfully integrated into the design of improved structures, rather than appended as a separate program. This is particularly important vis-à-vis STI treatment, harm reduction and substitution therapy for IDUs, and social and health service provision to uninsured, Roma, trafficked women, and other marginalized populations.

Macedonia. Macedonia has a relatively nascent epidemic; it should have sufficient fiscal and grant resources to manage both prevention and treatment approaches so that the epidemic does not spread. The Government should work across sectors (transportation, labor, education, and finance) to ensure a comprehensive approach to the problem. Government institutions need to ensure the development of public health infrastructure and HIV/AIDS interventions that are sustained beyond the implementation of the GFATM grant. In addition to addressing behavioral risks, particularly of youth, surveillance systems that detect, monitor, and evaluate the epidemic course within the highly vulnerable populations should be a priority activity, and linkages should be developed between other related programs, such as STI, TB control, reproductive health, prison health, and occupational health. Specifically, assistance may be required for:

- Coordination between different sectors, Ministries and services involved on HIV/AIDS, STIs and TB control has improved since the establishment of the Country Coordination Mechanism. The Parliament is considering decriminalization of CSW, but legislation regarding NGOs is necessary. Additional assistance is needed to further develop policy, and improve coordination. PLWHA should be included in the NMC; and the relative roles of the CCM and NMC have to be clarified.
- There is a need to strengthen public preventive services for vulnerable groups.
- As in other countries, surveillance needs to be established. However, this has not been included under the GFATM grant, so additional funding has to be identified for this activity.
- Monitoring and evaluation are being developed under the GFATM grant, but a M&E plan and indicators that allow for comparisons with other countries have to be adopted.
- The MOH needs technical assistance to manage the GFATM grant, and NGOs would welcome assistance and training on procurement and financial management. Mechanisms for transfer of funds from the GFATM grant to NGOs have to be established.

Serbia. In the short term, financial assistance is not necessary for many HIV/AIDS interventions, as the Government allocates significant funding to some prevention and treatment activities, and the country has obtained grants from the GFATM and DFID. However, technical support is necessary in the short term, and the country may need additional financial assistance in the short to medium term (3–5 years), as sustainability of the GFATM and DFID-funded programs may become an issue. Presently, the following areas need additional support:

- Establishing good coordination among different sectors and services involved on HIVAIDS, STIs and TB prevention and control.
- Supporting management of GFATM grant.
- Improving key public health functions such as surveillance, diagnosis and treatment of these diseases.
- Improving support to NGOs, including those involved on prevention and palliative care.

Montenegro. HIV/AIDS has been given a very low priority, due to the low number of registered cases, as well as competing priorities. It is only recently that Montenegro professionals started advocating among decisionmakers to strengthen the HIV/AIDS response. While the institutional capacity building and adapting functions of key government institutions present the initial challenge, a few broad-based AIDS prevention activities, including access to free HIV testing and counseling, public education, health promotion to modify risky sexual and drug using behaviors and effective harm reduction programs might have significant impact on prevention of HIV infection in Montenegro. Authorities may want to consider including a public health component under future health projects, which could respond to the local demand for further action on communicable diseases. The Institute of Public Health needs assistance in the following areas:

- Approval of an appropriate AIDS Strategy and preparation of a realistic GFATM grant proposal;
- Surveillance of communicable diseases, including HIV/AIDS; and
- Prevention and control of HIVAIDS, STIs and TB among youth, in prisons and among IDPs and Roma population.

Kosovo. Local authorities and NGOs should be supported to implement the approved HIV/AIDS Strategy. The substantial impact of the refugee situation in Kosovo, with the added impact of minority group discrimination should be addressed in any systematic approach to health system reform and HIV/AIDS prevention and control. These groups need special attention, and do not lend themselves to privatized, decentralized health system programs. In addition, the post-conflict trafficking and CSW situation needs a careful policy development approach that can be facilitated by interventions financed by the Bank on the health system or judicial system interventions. Public health activities such as surveillance systems and special studies on highly vulnerable populations and HIV prevention programs should be incorporated into health reform projects.

CHAPTER 5

The World Bank Role

The Bank has been focusing recently on ensuring an integrated regional approach to common challenges in ECA, including against HIV/AIDS. In South East Europe, the Bank has been cooperating in several regional programs, initiatives and studies, which either focus specifically on HIV/AIDS and populations vulnerable to HIV/AIDS, such as young people and trafficked people; or that may have an impact on the general context of risk referred to in this study.

The Bank's Role in South Eastern Europe

A *Regional Framework Paper for South Eastern Europe* is under preparation to provide a regional framework for the formulation of individual country assistance strategies, with the objective to ensure that programs have the greatest impact both at the country level and also at the regional level. The Strategy identifies areas of activity where there exist cross-border externalities or economies of scale, or opportunities for "scaling up" successful interventions across borders. It also identifies opportunities to encourage regional cooperation within the ambit of Bank activities, and provides a common path toward integration in European structures. Within this umbrella, the Bank has been collaborating on a variety of initiatives, including those mentioned below.

Studies

- Study on HIV/AIDS in the Western Balkans.
- The HIV/AIDS Study in South Eastern Europe, which includes case studies from Bulgaria, Croatia and Romania.

- The Study "Young People in South Eastern Europe: From Risk to Empowerment" provides a roadmap for youth development in SEE to assist governments, donors, and the World Bank with aligning public expenditures and investments with the needs and priorities of youth. The study outlines an integrated approach to the social, economic, and political participation of young people in society and identifies priority areas.
- The Study "Human Trafficking in South Eastern Europe: beyond crime control, and agenda for social inclusion and development" takes stock of current facts, contributing issues and responses to human trafficking in SEE.
- The Regional Study on Public Expenditure Policies in South Eastern Europe will highlight successful efforts to consolidate public expenditures and reduce the size of the state.
- "Building Market Institutions in South Eastern Europe: Comparative Prospects for Investment and Private Sector Development." This study was prepared in collaboration with EBRD. It carried out a review of institutional barriers to investment and growth in the eight SEE countries.
- Trade policies and institutions in the countries of South Eastern Europe in the EU stabilization and association process. This study reviews the economic performance of five Balkans countries—Albania, Bosnia and Herzegovina, Croatia, Macedonia, and Serbia and Montenegro—with a focus on international trade. It covers the current status regarding participation in the World Trade Organization (WTO), relations with the European Union (EU), and relations with each other, and other countries in Central and Eastern Europe.

Strategies

- A Regional Policy Note on Youth proposes options for action to reduce youth vulnerability including to HIV/AIDS, in the context of the Bank's policy dialogue, sector work and operations.
- A Framework for the Development of the Regional Transport System in the Balkans identifies and describes measures of regional importance that would promote trade in goods and in transport services among the Balkan countries and between these countries and the EU.
- A Regional Energy Strategy for the Balkans covering the South East Europe (SEE) regional energy market aims at contributing to increasing energy trade.

Initiatives

- The Social Development Initiative for South Eastern Europe aims at promoting the design of policies and programs that (i) support social cohesion through improved integration of ethnic minorities and youth as agents of social change and development, and (ii) reduce social tensions at the country and regional level. Advice to SEE governments and donors is provided in this process, and includes capacity building for institutions and for social analyses. The initiative has been supported by the Italian Development Co-operation and through the World Bank Post-Conflict Fund.

▨ The Bank continues to support selected regional initiatives under the Stability Pact, including the Infrastructure Working Group, Working Group on Trade Liberalization and Facilitation, the Investment Compact and the Anti-Corruption Initiative, in collaboration with the OECD and other partners.

▨ The Trade and Transport Facilitation Program for South Eastern Europe (TTFSE) aims to reduce non-tariff costs to trade and transport, to reduce smuggling and corruption at border crossings, and to strengthen customs and border control agencies in the region.

The Bank's Role on HIV/AIDS

The World Bank has had a significant role in prevention and control of HIV/AIDS globally, being one of the main sources of financing to fight the epidemic. The Bank is uniquely positioned to act simultaneously on risk factors and epidemic drivers that require short- and longer-term actions. The Bank provides technical and financial support to Governments to implement appropriate multi-sector strategies. It also supports country-led efforts through non-lending services as well as credits and loans. In addition, the Bank is a co-sponsor of the global coalition against HIV/AIDS—the Joint United Nations Program on HIV/AIDS (UNAIDS) and a Trustee of the Global Fund to Fight AIDS, Tuberculosis and Malaria (GFATM). These organizations work in partnership with governments, NGOs, bilateral organizations and multilateral agencies to support country and regional responses to HIV/AIDS.

Throughout the ECA region, Governments and civil society, in cooperation with international agencies and NGOs, have started working on developing HIV/AIDS Strategies and programs to respond to the challenge posed by the epidemic. The Bank has been working with a number of client countries and partner organizations in the region on assessing the situation and assisting the preparation and implementation of new interventions to address the challenges imposed by the HIV/AIDS epidemic. The Bank has been working with governments to secure commitments for effective actions, including political leadership and interventions through multisectoral approaches. The Bank has been partnering with UNAIDS, bilateral agencies and civil society groups to improve the knowledge base for HIV/AIDS work and catalyze a region-wide response to the epidemic.

Specifically, the Bank has had a role on HIV/AIDS prevention and control in ECA in the following areas:

▨ *Regional strategy.* The Bank has developed a regional strategy for the Bank work on HIV/AIDS in Europe and Central Asia (World Bank 2003a).

▨ *Regional sector work.* There are variations among countries in terms of the size of the epidemic, income per capita, the political contexts, infrastructure and management capacities. Therefore, the Bank has been carrying out analytical work in the ECA region to assess the HIV/AIDS situation and its potential human and economic impact, including part of Southeastern Europe: Bulgaria, Romania and Croatia (Novotny, Haazen, and Adeyi 2003), Georgia (Gotsadze, Chawla, and Chkatarashvili 2003), Poland and Baltic countries (Kulis and others 2003), and Central Asia (Godinho and others 2004, 2005).

■ *Estimating the economic impact of HIV/AIDS at the country level.* As mentioned before, this work has been carried out in Russia, Belarus, Moldova, and in Central Asia.

■ *Refining estimates of human and financial resources needs.* Local capacity for developing and implementing programs varies enormously. Available information indicates a substantial gap in the necessary resources for effective interventions on a large scale. Therefore, the Bank has co-financed with the UNAIDS Secretariat, the development of a Directory of Technical and Managerial Resources to enable countries to gain better access to high quality technical assistance; and a study of the incremental resource requirements for HIV/AIDS programs in ECA (UNAIDS and The World Bank 2003).

■ *Promoting a supportive policy environment.* With UNAIDS and other partners, the Bank is building support among key opinion leaders and elites for a dynamic HIV/AIDS control program. As this is particularly difficult due to the stigma attached (social, cultural, political), the Bank carried out public opinion research studies in Albania and the Kyrgyz Republic (Felzer 2004).

■ *Financing investments on HIV/AIDS control.* Given the relatively early stage of the epidemic, highest priority and Bank financing have been directed towards targeted interventions to prevent further transmission of the virus. In the Balkans, the Bank has supported HIV/AIDS activities through, for example, the Bosnia and Herzegovina Basic Health Project. In addition, the Bank is helping governments prepare projects that will support HIV/AIDS activities, as for example the Kosovo Youth Grant.

■ The Bank-financed AIDS Projects in ECA are the following:

● *The Moldova AIDS Control Project* supports the goal of Moldova's National Program for Prevention and Control of HIV/AIDS and STIs to reduce mortality, morbidity and transmission of HIV/AIDS, other sexually-transmitted infections and tuberculosis. The Project is a component of the national TB/AIDS Program, which is financed in parallel from the following grants: an IDA grant of US$5.5 million for AIDS, a USAID grant of US$4.0 million for TB, and a US$5.2 million grant from the Global Fund to Fight AIDS, TB and Malaria (GFATM), both for AIDS and TB. The Project is under satisfactory implementation.

● *The Russia TB and AIDS Control Project* ($150 million) supports the goal of the Government's Federal Program on Prevention and Control of Social Diseases to protect its population and economy from uncontrolled epidemics of TB, HIV/AIDS and other sexually-transmitted infections. The Project is under early implementation.

● *The Ukraine TB and HIV/AIDS Control Project* supports the Fourth Program on HIV/AIDS Prevention to reach the following objectives: to stabilize the epidemiological situation in the country; to reduce risky behavior among young people; and to reduce the social tension in the society and negative consequences of the epidemic. The total cost of the Project is $77 million, including a $60 million Bank loan, and $17 million from the Ukrainian government. The Project is under early implementation.

The Central Asia AIDS Control Project aims at contributing to decrease the potential epidemiological and economic impact of the epidemic in the region. The Project, which has been recently approved, is the first ECA regional project on HIV/AIDS. It involves Kazakhstan, Kyrgyz Republic, Tajikistan and Uzbekistan; and is financed by grants from IDA and DFID.

The Banks' Role on HIV/AIDS in the Western Balkans

In the Western Balkans, the Bank should continue to closely monitor the evolution of the HIV/AIDS epidemic, and gather more information about epidemic drivers; knowledge, attitudes and practices of most vulnerable groups and young people in general; cost-effectiveness of interventions that have worked in other regions; and potential impact of the epidemic on regional development. This evidence should inform Bank policy dialogue about AIDS in the region; and the inclusion of HIV/AIDS activities in Country Partnership and Poverty Reduction Strategies.

Taking into account that international aid is fading out in some of these countries; existing gaps in financing and technical assistance; and that sustainability of GFATM grants is uncertain in the medium term, the Bank may want to consider (i) increasing policy dialogue on prevention and control of HIV/AIDS and other communicable diseases such as STIs and tuberculosis; public health functions; and youth vulnerability; (ii) continuing sector work on HIV/AIDS and STIs; and (iii) investing on regional and country-specific operations that focus on decreasing youth vulnerability and improving public health functions that are key to preventing and controlling HIV/AIDS.

The Bank could play an important role in providing financial and technical assistance to the Balkans countries to prevent and control HIV/AIDS in the short to medium term. Areas of Bank assistance—actual and potential for the future—are indicated below.

- *Policy dialogue on implementation of approved HIV/AIDS Strategies.* This would include dialogue and technical assistance on:
  - Public health functions that are key to prevent and control HIV/AIDS, such as policy development, surveillance and prevention;
  - Institutional capacity to implement the approved strategies;
  - Resource allocations for prevention of HIV/AIDS;
  - Health care system requirements to treat people living with HIV/AIDS (PLWHA); and
  - Legislative and policy development to address highly vulnerable groups such as IDUs, MSM, CSW, prisoners and Roma populations.
- *Sector work on HIV/AIDS and STIs, drug use and commercial sex work, youth, and trafficking of human beings and drugs in the Balkans.* Regional counterparts in cooperation with the Bank and partner organizations should carry out further studies on HIV/AIDS and its drivers. The findings of this study suggest that it would be relevant to carry out the following studies in the near future:
  - Mapping movement of people and drugs in the Balkans;
  - Assessment of implementation capacity of public services and NGOs; and
  - In-depth resource review of public health expenditures (surveillance, prevention and control of communicable diseases), and resource needs.

Table 5. Areas of Bank Assistance (Actual and Potential)

	Policy dialogue	Sector work	Operations
Strategic and legal development	Assist regional Governments to finance and implement AIDS Strategies	Review of HIV/AIDS expenditures Update this study	Provide TA and financial support for strategic development under existing operations; and/or IDF Grants
Fund-raising & Management of funds	Assist CCMs in Albania, Bosnia and Herzegovina, Montenegro and Kosovo finalizing proposals to the GFATM	Update this study	Provide TA for fund-raising under existing operations and/or IDF grants
Surveillance	Advocate for investments in second generation surveillance	Update this study	To be included under possible future operation on AIDS and/or health
Prevention	Advocate for scaling up outreach activities with IDUs, CSWs, and prisoners	Update this study	To be included under possible future operation on AIDS and/or health and other sectors
Public Health	Advocate for investments in key public health functions	Carry out review of Public Health Services in the Balkans	To be included under possible future operations on health
Youth	Ongoing	Youth Study carried out	Kosovo Youth Grant under preparation

▨ *Training in leadership and decision-making, and HIV/AIDS expenditures review may* be provided by the World Bank Institute's Leadership Program on AIDS (LPA) for country counterparts.

▨ Options for possible Bank *financial and technical assistance for prevention and control of HIV/AIDS* in the short to medium term are indicated below.

    ● Include AIDS prevention and control components on poverty and sector operations.

    ● Develop operations that focus on decreasing youth vulnerability and improving public health functions that are key to prevent and control HIV/AIDS. Lessons learned from the proposed Kosovo Youth Development Post-Conflict Grant, which would include HIV/AIDS activities, may be valuable for the development of similar operations in a larger scale in other countries.

    ● IDA countries may want to apply for IDF grants and IDA grants for AIDS. IDF grants would finance updating the legal framework, and capacity building, including improving the fiduciary capacity of these countries to manage available HIV/AIDS funding. For example, the Kosovo Youth Project is expected to be financed by a Post-Conflict Grant. All countries may apply for Civil Society and Small Grants Programs. The Bank's Civil Society and Small Grants Program

might be encouraged to reach particularly vulnerable populations such as CSWs, homeless youth, Roma and migrants.
- A Regional Strategy to prevent and control HIV/AIDS in the Western Balkans may also be considered. This would cover the main transportation corridors in the Western Balkans. Similarly to the Regional AIDS operation that has been approved in Central Asia, such an operation could be co-financed by grants from IDA and partners that are active on HIV/AIDS in the Western Balkans.

CHAPTER 6

Profile: albania

Table 6. Epidemiology—Albania

Population	3.4 million
Registered HIV cases	148
Registered AIDS cases	48
IPH December 2004	
HIV/AIDS Prevalence Rate UNAIDS 2003	<0.1
New HIV Cases IPH 2003	2000–10
	2001–20
	2002–26
	2003–18
	2004–29
Modes of Transmission Euro-HIV 2003	66% Heterosexual
	10.4% MSM
	1.9% MTCT
	0.94% IDU
Registered STIs cases IPH 2003	Gonorrhea—6
	Syphilis—10
TB notification rate WHO	18 per 100,000

(*continued*)

Table 6. Epidemiology—Albania (*Continued*)

Vulnerable Groups	Youth
UNICEF 2002	▨ 60% under 34 of age are jobless
	▨ 56% of teenagers between 14–17 do not attend school
	▨ 15,000 abandoned children
	IDU
	▨ Over 30,000 IDUs
	▨ IDUs mean age: <21
	▨ 10–12% IDU prevalence among school-aged children
	▨ 73% of IDUs share needles
	▨ 85% of IDUs have never or only sometimes used condoms
	▨ 13% of IDUs are CSW
	▨ 20% of IDUs tested for HIV
	▨ 15% of IDUs always use condom
	CSW
	▨ Over 30,000 CSWs
	▨ 88% of CSW never or only sometimes use condoms
	▨ Some clients pay more to have sex without condoms
	▨ 80% of CSW have had an STI
	MSM
	▨ >70% HIV infected are male >10% infected through MSM
	▨ 15–28% of HIV/AIDS male cases reported having had sex with men

Epidemiological Overview

Although Albania entered the transition with a relatively healthy population, life expectancy has since fallen. Infant and under-five mortality rates remain relatively high, especially in rural areas, and maternal mortality is also high. The rates of contraception are low and those of abortion high. The prevalence of infectious diseases continues to be high, while that of chronic illnesses, such as cardiovascular disease (the leading cause of death), is rising. Several diseases preventable by vaccine are still common in Albania. There are also high rates of pulmonary TB and Hepatitis. While the number of cases of HIV/AIDS is still low, all risk factors that may lead to a rapid increase in the disease are present in Albania.

HIV Cases

Albania is currently ranked among countries with a low HIV/AIDS prevalence rate—the percentage of infected population is less than 0.1 percent. However, there are indications that the rate of infection is steadily increasing. The cumulative number of HIV registered cases by December 2004 was 148, of whom 48 have been diagnosed with AIDS. The number of notified cases of HIV is shown in Table 7. Over 70 percent of notified cases is thought to have acquired the infection abroad, which highlights the impact of migration on this

Table 7. HIV Notifications in Albania by Mode of Acquisition 1999–2004

	HIV Notifications					
Year	Total new cases (new cases in women)	Heterosexual	Homo-bisexual	Blood products	IDU	Vertical
1993	2					
1994	9					
1995	12					
1996	7					
1997	3					
1998	5					
1999	4					
2000	10 (3)	8	2	0	0	0
2001	20 (3)	16	4	0	0	0
2002	26 (10)	20	2	1	2	1
2003	21 (8)	10	2	0	0	3
2004	29 (10)	27	0	1	1	0
Total	148 (10)					

Source: Albania IPH

growing epidemic. The main mode of HIV transmission is sexual contact. In addition, prevalence of Hepatitis B and C antibodies among tested drug users is the highest in the region, at 65 percent and 18 percent respectively, indicating that sharing needles is a common practice.

Determining the extent and dynamics of HIV/AIDS in Albania is difficult. There has been no population-based, nationally representative serosurvey of HIV in the country. However, the reported HIV data may grossly underestimate the actual number of HIV infections, particularly given the country's weak HIV surveillance. Albania's National AIDS Program states that the number of reported HIV cases is only a small indication of the extent of the epidemic. Given the high percentage of HIV cases transmitted heterosexually, the percentage of female cases may be particularly under-reported. Most of the affected are in the age group 25–44 years of age.

Another factor in obtaining an accurate reflection of the situation is that different sources report different numbers. According to UNAIDS, in 1993, surveys (total n = 3,065) found that HIV prevalence was zero. However, no detail on the methodologies of these surveys is available (Hammers and Downs 2003). A UNICEF report (2002c) stated that as of the end of November 2001, there had been a cumulative total of 71 HIV infections reported in Albania, of which 82 percent were male. According to data presented at a 2002 regional HIV/AIDS conference—convened by USAID, DFID, UNAIDS, and the Government of Romania—93 percent of cumulative HIV infections reported were male and 73 percent were transmitted heterosexually (DFID 2002). In 1992, the Institute of Public Health in Tirana began reporting HIV/AIDS data to the European

Center for the Epidemiological Monitoring of AIDS (EuroHIV). EuroHIV (2003) reported that through the end of June 2003, Albania had reported a cumulative total of 106 HIV infections. However, this figure represents only reported infections, 70 (66.0 percent) were transmitted heterosexually, 11 (10.4 percent) via MSM, 2 (1.9 percent) through mother-to-child transmission, and 1 (0.9 percent) via IDU. However, EuroHIV did not provide data on transmission via unsafe blood/blood products nor on gender distribution.

AIDS Cases and Deaths

According to data from the IPH, through the end of 2004, there had been a cumulative total of 48 AIDS cases reported in Albania. Among those cases for which transmission mode was identified, 30 cases (81 percent) were transmitted heterosexually, and 3 cases (8 percent) via MSM. No cases via IDU or MTCT were reported.

Sexually-transmitted Infections

Officially reported cases of sexually-transmitted diseases in Albania are very low: in 2000, there were 6 cases of gonorrhea and, in 1999, there were 10 cases of syphilis. Prior to the 1950s, however, Albania had endemic syphilis, as did many other countries in the region. A complex strategy for syphilis control and prevention was initiated throughout the country in the 1950s, leading to a sharp decrease in syphilis during the 1960s and a reported elimination of syphilis during the 1972–1994 period. This is consistent with very low rates of syphilis notification reported in most western European countries during the 1970s and 1980s. Rates of notification of syphilis per 100,000 population between 1960 and 2002 are shown in Figure 5.

Rates of notification of gonorrhea per 100,000 population between 1960–2002 are shown in 1.1. There has been a more or less continuous decline in notifications since 1984, with only 2 cases notified in 2001. There is no reliable notification or surveillance system for chlamydia infection. However, data on prevalence of chlamydia is available from

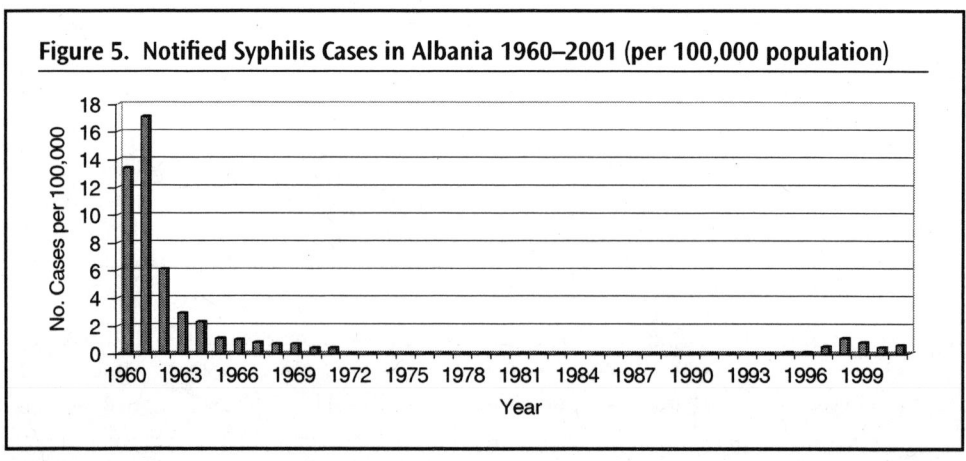

Figure 5. Notified Syphilis Cases in Albania 1960–2001 (per 100,000 population)

Source: Albania IPH.

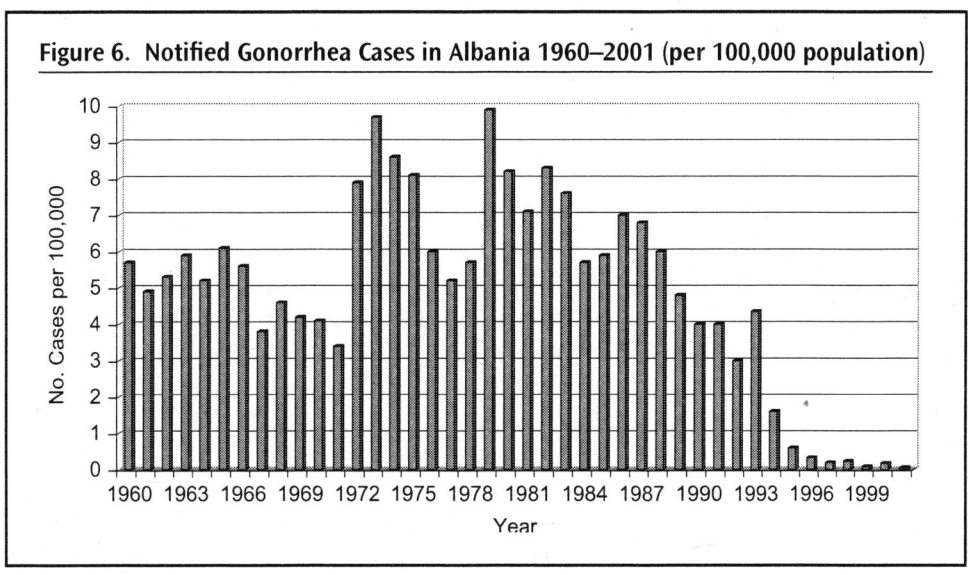

Figure 6. Notified Gonorrhea Cases in Albania 1960–2001 (per 100,000 population)

Source: Albania IPH.

cross-sectional surveys among 384 gynecological outpatients and inpatients in 2001 and 2002. Chlamydia prevalence in this group was 12–13 percent.

The re-emergence of STIs in Albania in the mid-1990s, specifically syphilis, may reflect a complex series of influences, including decreased effectiveness of control mechanisms, increased migration and commercial sex work, and changes to patterns of sexual partner formation. It is likely that the true rates of incident cases during the re-emergence of the infection are considerably higher than the notification rate. This is because the notification system has become less effective. More people now seek health care in the private sector, yet it is the public health care system that officially tracks STIs. Similarly, the rapid decline of gonorrhea during the early 1990s could also point to a decline in the effectiveness of the notification system. Low rates of gonorrhea during the late 1990s—when syphilis was increasing—undoubtedly indicate that the vast majority of cases are not obtaining care within the public health care system. Given the re-emergence of syphilis, it is unlikely that gonorrhea rates dropped from 149 per 100,000 population in the period of 1972 to 1994, to 8 per 100,000 reported thereafter.

Vulnerability to HIV/AIDS: Contextual Factors

In 2003, Albania's population was about 3.4 million people (U.S. Department of State 2003a). Albania is far more rural (54 percent) than other countries in Southern Europe (30 percent; PRB 2003). Its inhabitants are 95 percent Albanian, 3 percent Greek, and the remainder is Vlach, Roma, Serb, Montenegrin, Macedonian, Egyptian, and Bulgarian. About 70 percent of the population is Muslim, 20 percent Albanian Orthodox, and 10 percent Roman Catholic.

Albania shares a frontier with Greece to the south/southeast, Macedonia to the east, and Serbia and Montenegro to the north and northeast. The coastline of western Albania lies along the Adriatic and Ionian seas. The country's primary seaport is Durres, which handles 90 percent of its maritime cargo. Since 1993, Albania has been divided into

---

Table 8. Vulnerability Factors—Albania

GNI per Capita World Bank 2001	US$1,340
Unemployment UNICEF 2001	15%
Poverty GFATM proposal 2004	30%
Mobility GFATM proposal 2004	▓ More than 70% reported HIV cases are among young men who have contracted the disease while abroad
Trafficking IOM 2001	▓ Migration rate—10.4 per 1000 people
	▓ 43% of Albania youth are migrant workers
	▓ 350,000 migrant workers abroad (20% of the labor force)
	▓ High internal, rural-to-urban migration
	▓ 30,000 Albanian women from rural areas increasingly work as CSW abroad
	▓ 14% of victims of trafficking in Italy are Albanian nationals
	▓ Albania is one of the main transit countries for trafficking Eastern European women to the west

---

12 administrative areas called prefectures, each comprising an average of three districts with one central administration. Each district has at least one municipality and several communes; there are 315 communes and 42 municipalities in the country. Although, in theory, they all have the power to collect taxes, in practice local governments receive most of their annual revenue from the central government.

Albania was a communist state from 1944 until 1991. During this period, its isolation and lack of export earnings contributed to its underdevelopment and persistent poverty. Since the fall of communism in Eastern Europe, the transition from centralized government to a more developed free market economy has had an intense, disruptive impact on the population.

During the initial transition period, the government introduced basic democratic reforms, including a multi-party system. However, economic and democratic reform slowed in the mid-1990s. The crisis of 1997, followed by the 1999 Kosovo crisis, caused a severe economic recession, which resulted in high unemployment and a weakened health and education infrastructure (UNFPA and PRB 2003). Between 1997–2002, a series of short-lived governments succeeded one another.

The government has taken measures to curb violent crime and to revive economic activity and trade. Traditional kinship links in Albania, centered on the patriarchal family, are being shattered by the transition to an open, modern market economy, industrialization, and internal migration from the countryside to urban areas. The 2001 UNDP gender-related development index ranked Albania the lowest in Eastern Europe.

Economy

Albania has made significant progress since its transition to a market economy. The democratically elected government that assumed office in April 1992 launched an ambitious economic reform program. Initially, results were encouraging, but in 1995, progress stalled. The collapse of the pyramid schemes in 1997 and the civil unrest that followed were a major setback, from which Albania's economy continues to recover.

Despite periods of domestic and regional instability, Albania has achieved high growth while containing inflation. However, the country faces enormous challenges. Although GNI per capita has risen, Albania remains one of the poorest countries in Europe (World Bank 2003j). Unemployment is high, particularly among young people; according to UNICEF, 60 percent of those under age 34 do not have a job (Wong 2002a). Weak and deteriorating infrastructure and services throughout the country left 40 percent of households without reliable access to basic education, water, sanitation, and heating, and only the capital of Tirana can depend on uninterrupted electrical power. The country faces concurrent challenges to reduce poverty, improve employment opportunities, attract foreign investment, improve transparency in business procedures, restructure the banking and tax systems, reduce corruption, resolve property ownership disputes, ensure the rule of law, improve social services, and address a precarious energy situation.

Agriculture accounts for approximately 34 percent of Albania's GDP, followed by the service sector (32 percent), remittances from Albanian workers abroad (mostly in Greece and Italy) (21 percent), and industry (13 percent). Two-thirds of all workers are employed in the agriculture sector, although the construction and service industries have been expanding. Although certain sectors provide severely needed economic opportunities—transport, tourism, and mining, as well as the high dependence on remittances from abroad—these sectors also entail an increase in mobility, possible regroupings of family units, and exposure to new sexual networks, all of which may have significant ramifications for HIV transmission. In addition, informal labor markets play an important role in Albania's economy, a scenario that will affect government and civil society's ability to reach Albanians through workplace HIV/AIDS interventions.

Poverty

Albania is one of the poorest countries in Europe, with 2001 GNI per capita of US$1,340. One-fourth of the Albanian population is poor. Extreme poverty is low, at less than 5 percent of the population, but many families live close to the poverty line. Poverty is higher in rural areas and more prevalent among young families. Among the key findings of the country's 2002 Living Standards Measurement Survey are the following:

- Almost half of the poor in Albania are under 21 years of age.
- The north and northeastern regions are among the poorest in the country.
- The poor and extremely poor have a low coefficient of school registration, particularly high school registration.
- The poor benefit less from health services.
- The unemployment rate among the poor is about twice as high as that of the non-poor.
- Among poor families, the main source of income is agricultural activity and salaried employment.
- The poor spend over half their income on food (67 percent).

Mobility

More than 70 percent of reported HIV cases are among young men residing abroad, who have reported that they contracted the disease while abroad. Many Albanian adults seek work far from home, mostly due to economic pressures. The net migration rate is 10.4 per 1,000 people, which represents 350,000 migrant workers abroad (20 percent of the labor force). Of the nearly 750,000 people who have left between 1990 and 1999, nearly 70 percent are males 16–30 years old (ICMH 2000). Almost one-third of young adults have spent some time working abroad. There are generally three types of young people who move abroad: (1) long-term emigrants; (2) seasonal or temporary emigrants (including tourists); and (3) students. Data from a survey of Albanians living in Greece and Italy indicated that the main reasons for emigration were: higher wages, better working conditions, better living standards, better educational opportunities, ability to provide financial assistance to families still living in Albania, and political reasons (Wong 2002a).

Albania has the highest residential instability in the region. Since restrictions on freedom of movement were lifted in the 1990s, there has been a dramatically high level of internal migration from rural to urban areas. In 1979, only 33.5 percent of the population was urban; by 2001, this figure had reached 46 percent. Because of this influx, the population in the region of Tirana has increased rapidly to over 500,000, with concomitant strains on infrastructure and health services. Intracountry migration has also contributed to an increased level of conflict and crime in urban areas. Another major population shift occurred in early 1999, when over 700,000 people fled Kosovo, with about 450,000 Kosovars seeking refuge in Albania. However, fewer than 300 of these refugees now remain in Albania (Refugees International 2003a).

Vulnerable Groups

Although extended family ties in Albania weakened during the political and economic transition, they are still strong, to the point that relatives still care for most dependent older people. In general, however, there are no or few services at the community level for vulnerable groups, including at-risk children and youth, mobile populations, women, sex workers, illicit drug users, MSM, and ethnic minorities. Women may have unique vulnerabilities in Albania. According to UNDP (2003):

> "Women suffer from diminished political and economic opportunities and, at the same time, play a reduced role in community decision making. Men seem to have more ready access to jobs than women; the sudden drop in access to public child-care facilities and the consequent greater burdens of child care and unemployment have affected women more than men."

Youth. Albania's population is on average younger than that of other European countries—32 percent of the population is under age 15. In 2000, the country's median age was 26.7 (UNAIDS 2003e). The Bank study on Young People in SEE found that young males are especially vulnerable to social and economic exclusion (Cava and others 2004). According to Albania's 1999 KAPB survey, health was the most important challenge mentioned with regard to children, followed by education and economic opportunities. According to UNICEF (2000), 90 percent of children of primary school age attend primary school. The majority (88 percent) of the population over age 15 is literate (UNICEF 2000), although there are disparities between urban (93 percent) and rural areas (81 percent). However, since the transition began, gross enrollment rates for basic and secondary education have declined. Schools in urban areas are overcrowded, school dropout rates are high (particularly in rural areas), and illiteracy among the younger age groups is increasing. UNICEF reports that only 39 percent of youth ages 14–17 attend high school. This low rate is a result of "declining interest in school" (which could be due to high unemployment and the perception that the economic return on an education is low, which, to a large extent, is correct), as well as emigration and migration within the country. Moreover, the underfunded education system has been unable to respond effectively to the needs of mobile populations arriving in coastal areas and large urban areas.

Women. According to a 2000 report from Albania's National Committee of Women and Family and UNICEF, the incidence of domestic violence has become worse in the last ten years. Domestic violence in Albania remains clandestine and is supported by the traditional and patriarchal attitude in the Kanun (code of customary laws used in the northern part of Albania). Alcoholism, jealousy, unemployment, and poverty are cited as among the main causes. The higher level of economic dependency of women, the absence of law enforcement, and the lack of legislative protection for women inside and outside the home all contribute to the cycle of violence. Only 5 percent of cases of domestic violence are brought to court. Many journalistic reports on domestic violence victimize the abused woman and reinforce existing prejudices and stereotypes. NGO efforts include lobbying for human rights, organizing public awareness campaigns on the issue, and offering services and support to abused women, girls, and children.

Crime has increased substantially during the transition period, but the government has taken measures to reduce violent crime. Data from the U.N. Office on Drugs and Crime (2002) indicate that the number of criminal convictions in Albania has been rising, which may be the result of improved law enforcement and efficiencies of the judiciary system.

Trafficked People. Human trafficking is one of the country's most serious problems. Albania is a source and transit country primarily for women and children trafficked for sexual exploitation and begging, respectively. These women come from all parts of Albania, although increasingly, they come from rural areas. Most of them are ages 20 to 24 years. Women are trafficked to Italy and Greece, and on to other EU countries, such as Belgium, France, the U.K., and the Netherlands. Victims transitting Albania primarily come from Romania and Moldova, with smaller numbers from Bulgaria and Ukraine. Children are also reportedly trafficked from Albania to work as beggars in Italy and Greece. According to the U.S. Department of State (2003d), although the Government of Albania does not meet the minimum standards for the elimination of trafficking—hindered by, among other factors, corruption and lack of protection for vulnerable children—it is making significant efforts to do so.

Sex Workers. Exploitation of prostitution and the increase in commercial sex work present a risk for the spread of HIV/AIDS, especially if taking into consideration the low rate of condom use. As many as 30,000 Albanian women and girls might be working as commercial sex workers in Europe (UNICEF 2002c). Over the past 12 years, thousands of Albanian women have worked in the sex industry in Western Europe and other Balkan countries.

Many of these women have been trafficked for sex work, either through false promises of marriage or employment, or through coercion at the time of kidnapping. Although prostitution is illegal in Albania, women are often forced into sex work while waiting to leave Albania. Albania's 1999 KAPB survey found that there may be a growing acceptance of sex work as a livelihood.

Children, including boys, are also victims of sexual trafficking. Deported children have often been arrested abroad as illegal migrants and kept in detention centers together with traffickers and other adult illegal migrants, where they are often abused by guards or other inmates (UNICEF 2002c). Most of the children at risk of trafficking for labor and prostitution are members of ethnic minorities and are increasingly from rural areas. A report by the Albanian government states that approximately 5,000 children are victims of criminal networks in child exploitation and trafficking. Some official estimates show that 70 percent of Albanians who claim disability benefits are young people under the age of 18. Further, the number of social orphans is rising (children from families in crisis, abandoned by their parents); 15,000 children have been abandoned by one or both parents since the transition began.

MSM. The Albania GFATM proposal (2004) estimates that 2 percent of the male population would be homosexual, which represents 35,000 people. Although homosexual behavior is not prosecuted since 1995, the MSM community is still highly stigmatized and experiences a high level of discrimination. Police interrogate and detain Albanian gay people frequently. Consequently, it has been difficult for the Albanian homosexual community to organize itself socially and politically, and to gain access to existing services. The Albanian Lesbians and Gays Association was recently established, but its activities remain limited. Sex work has emerged as a strategy of survival for some Albanian men who emigrate to Greece and Italy, many of whom return to Albania.

Drug Users. Though few HIV cases have been detected among drug users, future expansion of the epidemic may take place mostly among IDUs, following the pattern observed in other countries in the region. Estimates vary, but it appears that there may be up to 30,000 illicit drug users in Albania. According to UNAIDS, 70 percent of Albania's drug users inject. In 1997–1998, the prevalence of drug use among school-aged children was between 10–12 percent. Drug use appears to be highest among Roma youth, who represent 60 percent of the 12–13 age group. The most commonly used drugs are cannabis, cocaine, and heroin. Cannabis users represents the majority of drug users, while heroin and cocaine users represent 10–25 percent of all drug users, although this group reflects a high prevalence of risk behaviors such as sharing equipment and having unprotected sex. Based on treatment demand data, drug injecting is increasing (27 percent of drug users seeking treatment in 1999 were IDUs, compared to 19.5 percent just a year earlier). At the Tirana Toxicological Clinic, IDUs comprised 80 percent during the first half of 2001. In addition to serving as a transit point for cocaine and heroin, Albania also produces cannabis (mainly concentrated in south). Trafficking and production of drugs have been spreading rapidly throughout Albania; factors that contribute to this include: conflict in the region, lack of preparedness to address drug issues, weak law enforcement, increased population mobility, poverty, high unemployment, and lack of economic and socio-cultural opportunities for young people.

Table 9. UNICEF Rapid Assessment—Albania[6]

Study site

Tirana: capital city, with highest number of inhabitants (over half a million) and highest number of illicit drug users (estimated at 8,000)	▓ The main drug used is heroin, but cannabis is most often the first illicit drug consumed by DUs. ▓ Injecting drug use is increasing (65%) and the level of needle/syringe sharing is high (74%). ▓ The sexual risk behaviors of drug users are also high. Over two-thirds (78%) do not always use a condom. Over 30% have had two to five sexual partners in the last year. ▓ Interviewed drug users considered themselves relatively informed on HIV/AIDS; however, the accuracy of their knowledge on certain issues was poor, as was knowledge of STIs and hepatitis. Some drug treatment centers, harm reduction centers (needle exchange), and rehabilitation centers exist; however, these interventions need to enhance their services to meet increased demand.
Shkodra: relatively large, young population bordering Montenegro, considered a transit point and trafficking route of women and drugs; evidence of drug production (cannabis) and increasing number of drug users	▓ Cannabis and heroin are the main drugs used. (Heroin users progressively switch from smoking to injecting.) ▓ Approximately 77% percent of drug users inject. Over two-thirds of injectors share needles and/or syringes (74%). ▓ Over half of drug users have had six to ten sexual partners in the last year. Only 3% of respondents always use a condom; 81% have had sexual intercourse under the influence of drugs. ▓ There is a low level of awareness and knowledge of HIV/AIDS and other STIs. Personal perception of HIV/STIs risk is low. Few drug users have been tested for HIV. ▓ There is no intervention (prevention, harm reduction, rehabilitation or treatment) targeting drug users in Shkodra. Information, education, and communication activities regarding illicit drugs are scarce.
Vlora: port city considered a transit point for trafficked women and girls to Western countries (via speedboats to Italy)	▓ Sex work is closely linked with trafficking of women and girls. ▓ Condom use is very low. ▓ Awareness and knowledge of HIV/AIDS/STIs is low. ▓ Although a high proportion of sex workers considered themselves at risk of contracting HIV/STIs, this self-perception rarely resulted in changed behavior. ▓ About 80% of sex workers report having had an STI. ▓ Many sex workers report physical and mental abuse from clients or protectors. ▓ Sex workers do not view health care services as easily accessible, nor do they perceive these services to be friendly/open to them and their special needs. Existing interventions involve just NGOs, which mainly provide some psychosocial support, legal assistance, and short-term shelter for repatriated sex workers.

(*continued*)

---

6. UNICEF RAR October 2001–January 2002. Fieldwork for this study was undertaken between October 2001 and January 2002 and data were collected from participants ages 10–24 (n = 314) in four sites: Tirana, Shkodra, Vlora, and Korça.

Table 9. UNICEF Rapid Assessment—Albania[6] (*Continued*)

Study site

Korça: border city close to Greece experiencing a high level of population mobility
- Main factors driving emigration among youth are economic, although tourism and education also come into play.
- Almost 90% of young people interviewed have had sexual intercourse, with about half having had two to five partners during the last year.
- Condom use is quite low.
- There is a lack of accurate knowledge and awareness on HIV/AIDS/STIs.

Data from a UNICEF's Rapid Assessment (Chart 1) are useful in understanding young people's vulnerability to acquiring HIV, particularly given the general lack of data on HIV/AIDS awareness, knowledge, and risk behaviors. However, as UNICEF itself states, caution should be used in extrapolating the findings regarding the general youth population.

Prisoners. As of June 2003, none of the reported HIV/AIDS cases was among prisoners. However, little is known about the epidemiological situation of HIV and STIs within the prisons. No mandatory HIV testing is required for prisoners. The only available data for risky behaviors among prisoners come from a survey conducted by the NGO "STOP AIDS." Use of alcohol and drugs is forbidden inside the prison system. There are ten prisons in Albania with an average of 2,600 prisoners. However, Albania has been asked to receive 4,000 Albanian prisoners who are presently serving time in Greece, Italy and Switzerland (Albania 2004).

Roma. Poverty among Roma remains one of the most pressing issues for Central and Eastern Europe. The Roma population is considered an underprivileged ethnic minority, with lower socio-economic status, and is considered more vulnerable to HIV in comparison to the general population. Discrimination and low social cohesion contribute to poor education, and also to a lack of access to preventive services messages and other efforts geared towards the general population. Two-thirds of young Roma interviewed in the context of

---

Table 10. Knowledge, Attitudes and Practices—Albania

Knowledge	25% of all women know 3 ways how to prevent HIV transmission
UNICEF 1999, 2000	77% of all women do not know where to obtain an HIV test
	33% of men have ever used condom
	12% of CSW always use condoms
Practices	74% of men consider the price reasonable
UNICEF 2000	47% IDUs have between 2–5 sex partners per year
	62% of CSW have between 50–99 sex partners per year
	30% of CSW have over 100 sex partners per year

UNICEF's Rapid Assessment were illiterate and only 3 percent of them perceived themselves to be at risk for HIV or STIs. UNICEF reported in 2000 that two-thirds of the children living or working on the streets were of the Roma minority group. These children are involved in begging and/or sex work, which results in increased sexual partners and higher rates for use of drugs, including injecting drugs. Roma also test at higher proportionate rates for HIV because many are paid blood donors.

HIV/AIDS Awareness and Knowledge

The MISC survey[7] found that only 25 percent of women ages 15–49 knew all three important ways to prevent HIV transmission. Misconceptions about HIV/AIDS are high. For example, only 12.6 percent stated that mosquitoes cannot spread AIDS (among women ages 15–24, this figure is 14 percent); 77 percent did not know where to obtain an HIV test; and only 0.7 percent has been tested for HIV. Among the findings, only 12 percent of women ages 15–24 and 9 percent ages 25–49 expressed a positive attitude toward people living with HIV/AIDS.

Albania's 1999 KAPB survey reflects that approximately one-third of the 1,041 respondents mentioned AIDS as the main health problem facing Albania today. Over half of the respondents were under the age of 30; 70 percent lived in urban districts. Only 6 percent of the people ages 46–50 referred to AIDS. Most people replied that they had heard about HIV/AIDS from television. Generally, a large proportion of the survey population, especially younger people, said they were very or moderately worried about getting HIV/AIDS, and 194 people said they had friends or relatives who they thought should change their behavior to avoid getting the disease.

Even in the youngest age group, 15–20 years old, 19 percent said they knew someone who should take action to avoid getting HIV/AIDS. Regardless, 14 percent of people in the youngest age group said they had never talked with relatives about the problem and another 17 percent said they had probably spoken about it no more than "once or twice." Although awareness of HIV/AIDS was high, there were numerous misconceptions about how HIV is transmitted. For example, respondents believed the following practices to be very or moderately risky in HIV transmission: shaking hands (26 percent); having sex with someone with HIV/AIDS even with a condom (69 percent); using public toilets (more than 60 percent); donating blood (83 percent); and receiving a blood transfusion (96 percent).

The 1999 KABP survey found that knowledge about condoms was good, but use was low. Over 82 percent of the men in the survey said they knew what a condom was. This was particularly evident in the 15–30 year-old age group. However, only 33 percent of men said they had ever used one, most of whom were in the 21–30 year-old age group, suggesting that the popularity of condoms is a relatively recent phenomenon. Men who had completed high school and lived in the main urban areas were by far more likely than others to use condoms, but even so, only 9 percent of them said they had used one the last time they had sex. The price of condoms was clearly not a problem; 74 percent of the men who purchased condoms said the price was reasonable; another 23 percent said they thought it was low. Approximately 27 percent said they liked condoms because they were easy to find and

---

7. Albania Multiple Indicator Cluster Survey (MICS) 1999. UNICEF. The MICS survey used interviews carried out in household clusters (n = 5,000) to be nationally representative.

Box 13: Public Opinion Research in Albania

Opinion leaders and the general public:

- Do not regard HIV/AIDS as requiring immediate attention
- Welcome outside groups (international NGOs, multi/bi-laterals) to work on HIV/AIDS
- Believe that the basic health infrastructure is of much more pressing importance than HIV/AIDS
- Are highly aware of the HIV/AIDS issue yet there are information gaps

Opportunities and Obstacles:

- Growing openness in Albanian society provides an excellent opportunity to bring frank discussions in the public arena
- But conservative and traditional attitudes still prevalent
- Resistance to condom use
- Opinion leaders very conscious of Albania's reputation while general public more conscious about value of education
- Great support for educational campaigns (esp. in schools) however no trust in school officials
- Crucial to pierce the sense of invulnerability that most people (including young people) have with regard to HIV/AIDS and to aggressively promote safe sex and condom usage

---

Source: Felzer 2004.

36 percent said that good advertising had brought two specific brands to their attention. The majority of drug users and commercial sex workers do not use condoms when they have sex.

The UNICEF Rapid Assessment (UNICEF 2002c; Baran 2002) included a sample of emigrants. Among sexually active emigrants (89 percent of the total) 40 percent had sex with a sex worker abroad; 82 percent did not always use a condom, and almost 50 percent stated "not liking sex with condom" as a reason. Many emigrants do not seek health services abroad for fear of being expelled (illegal immigrants) or due to the lack of information on laws or rights of immigrants. The main source of information on HIV/AIDS was television (30 percent and 33 percent of respondents, respectively; WHO 2001).

A 1999 national survey of Albanians found that in response to questions concerning the main health problems facing the country, approximately one-third of respondents mentioned AIDS (ICMH 2002). However, high-level political commitment to addressing HIV/AIDS, financing needed interventions, and acutely needed planning, priority setting, and programs remains lacking.

In 2003, the Bank carried out a qualititative poll of selected opinion leaders and a quantitative survey of 1,000 people nationwide, aged 15–59, to check the level of awareness and attitudes regarding HIV/AIDS in the country. The main results of this study are presented in the box below.

Health Care in Albania

In general, health care in Albania has been a low priority. Health services are particularly poor in rural areas, where the majority of the population lives. The health care system continues to face serious structural, managerial, and financial challenges. Consequently, the quality and quantity of health care services, including accessibility remains problematic.

Existing services for vulnerable populations have limited capacity and geographic coverage, thereby excluding many in rural and isolated communities. The Bank-financed Health Projects have been addressing some of these constraints.

The Ministry of Health (MOH) began a process of health sector reform. The MOH identified two overarching objectives: prevent further deterioration of basic services and transform the health care system into a financially sustainable system that can be managed efficiently and produce effective services. MOH is the major financier and provider of health care services in Albania. The Ministry assumes the lead role in most areas of health care. It owns most health services, with the partial exception of primary care. The Ministry dedicates most of its efforts to health care administration, and only recently is gradually assuming a national policy-making and planning role.

A crucial area of the government's health sector reform is decentralization. However, the health care system remains highly centralized and hierarchical. Some administrative responsibility (but no political or policy responsibility) has been devolved to the 12 newly created regional prefectures. The MOH intends to test various models before proceeding with a larger decentralization program. Decentralization has not been accompanied by a clear definition of responsibilities. Various government entities often lack the political will to discharge their duties, and sometimes do not understand the new rules and regulations. Thus, according to a 2002 report from the European Observatory on Health Care Systems, there is tension between the various stakeholders, and central legislative bodies sometimes pass contradictory regulatory acts given these divergent interests, thus creating more confusion.

Social health insurance was introduced in 1995. The Health Insurance Institute (HII) is a quasi-governmental body accountable to the Parliament. Coverage was extended since 1996, and individual contributions to the national fund are, in principle, compulsory.

The Institute of Public Health (IPH) is responsible for public health, particularly for monitoring, prevention, and control of infectious diseases, and environmental health. The IPH works mainly through the district public health services. In 2000, the IPH merged with the former National Directorate of Health Education and Promotion, and it now assumes the directorate's former functions.

The Primary Health Care (PHC) network is not fully utilized, especially by people living close to urban areas. In addition, lack of sufficient funds and supervision prevents the centers from being in good operating condition and providing quality services. MOH has begun to integrate other health services into PHC teams. As part of this process, TB prevention services will become part of primary care, as will public health and preventive services such as school health, health education, MCH services, and family planning. The country now has 51 hospitals, including specialist hospitals and a military hospital. Albania's ratio of hospital beds to population is among the lowest in Europe. Tertiary care remains very limited and is located mainly in Tirana by the following facilities: Tirana University Hospital (also called Mother Tereza), with about 1,600 beds, the largest hospital in the country, Tirana Obstetric and Gynecology Hospital, Lung Disease Hospital, offering long-term treatment for TB patients, and Military Hospital, under the Ministry of Defense.

Private health services reappeared in Albania in the early 1990s. Most private services are provided in diagnostic centers and specialized outpatient clinics and located in large urban areas, particularly Tirana. As yet, there are no private hospitals or inpatient facilities in Albania. Most private sector facilities are well equipped and organized. Some of these

Table 11. Health Expenditure and GDP Trends in Albania 1990–2001

Albania	1990	1995	1996	1997	1998	1999	2000	2001
Health expenditure per capita (current US$)		26	31	23	33	40	41	
Health expenditure, public (% of GDP)	3.35	2.54	2.45	2.04	2.1	2.18	2.3	2.0
GDP per capita, PPP (current international $)	2,605	2,612	2,915	2,736	2,939	3,226	3,541	3,738
GDP growth (annual %)	−9.58	8.9	9.1	−7	7.87	7.25	7.8	6.48

Source: World Bank HNP Statistical Database.

health services are financed and organized by foreign NGOs, private agencies, or religious bodies. However, there are no mechanisms in place to monitor the quality of services offered by private facilities, nor are there links between private and public facilities.

Albania has few trained health care professionals in comparison to other European countries. Moreover, the distribution of health care professionals remains concentrated in hospitals (as in most countries with a Soviet model health care system). In addition, there are large disparities in number of staff among different districts. These imbalances are mainly the result of the difficult living and working conditions in remote rural areas. Albania is also experiencing a severe brain drain. During 1990–1999, an estimated 40percent of professors and researchers at Albanian universities and research centers left the country.

Most of the pharmaceutical distribution system in Albania is private. About 12 wholesale companies import most of the drugs, biologic products, and diagnostic equipment in the country. A network of about 750 private pharmacies and pharmaceutical agencies ensure drug distribution across the country. The two state pharmaceutical manufacturers, Profarma and the Antibiotics Factory, have been privatized. The country's 500 plus private pharmacies are well stocked and better managed than hospital dispensaries. Although there is sufficient supply of essential drugs, the absence of a good regulatory framework allows poor practices to continue such as the dispensing of drugs that are of inferior quality, outdated, or unregistered.

Funding of Health Services

Financing levels for Albanian health care remain very low; moreover, the proportion of financing through out-of-pocket expenditures has been increasing, which has raised concerns about equitable access to health care. Public expenditure for health accounted for 2.2 percent of the GDP, or 7 percent of total public expenditure in 2002. Although these figures represent an increase from 2 and 6 percent, respectively, in 2001, provision of resources for the health sector in Albania is still unsatisfactory.

Health services in Albania are funded from mainly two sources, tax-financed government contributions to the sector and a statutory health insurance scheme. In addition, foreign aid contributed around 3 percent of total health financing in 2003. This funding system suffered from dwindling resources over the last couple of years, mainly caused by

Table 12. Government Intervention and Institutional Arrangements—Albania

Intersectoral coordination	▦ National HIV/AIDS Committee is chaired by the Vice-Prime Minister
	▦ GFATM Country Coordination Mechanism (CCM) has been established
National HIV/AIDS Strategy and Legislation	▦ Strategy paper "Policies of Prevention and Control of HIV/AIDS/STI Epidemic in Albania" not yet approved
	▦ National AIDS Program is developed by IPH but without clear priorities
	▦ Law on Reproductive Health was approved in 2002
Government institution responsible for HIV/AIDS	▦ The Institute of Public Health (IPH) leads the National Program for HIV/AIDS. It is recognized as the national reference laboratory and center of expertise for HIV testing and diagnosis
	▦ Ministry of Public Order and UNODC undertaking capacity building in anti-drug police unit (drug law enforcement and HIV primary prevention)
National AIDS Program	▦ Until recently was staffed only by 2 people, although the government recently allocated funds to enlarge activities. It is supposed to coordinate with other ministries and government institutions

a very weak tax base, the low-income levels, and a large informal sector. Although the state is still the main source of health care funding, public funding decreased from around 84 percent in 1990 to less than 40 percent in 2003. This has led to equity and access problems for the poor and vulnerable population groups without insurance coverage, as well as for rural populations. In-patient services, including tuberculosis treatment, are free of charge for the whole population, but quality of care is often low.

With regard to HIV/AIDS, no detailed information was available on the structure and amount of financing for specific HIV/AIDS-related activities in Albania.

Government and Civil Society Action on HIV/AIDS

The HIV/AIDS Strategic, Policy, and Regulatory Framework

A National AIDS Conference entitled "Policies of Prevention and Control of HIV/AIDS/STI Epidemic in Albania" was held in 1998. A strategy paper was produced. A National AIDS Committee has been established, chaired by the vice Prime Mnister, to lead and coordinate national efforts to combat HIV/AIDS. The process of drafting the National Strategy, was supported by a number of international and local stakeholders. However, the National AIDS Committee rarely meets, indicating the low government commitment to HIV/AIDS. A GFATM Country Coordination Mechanism (CCM) has been formally established to apply for a grant, but appears to be ineffective. Due to competing priorities in the fast economic adjustment and low prevalence of HIV, the Poverty Reduction Strategy Paper (PRSP) does not take HIV/AIDS as a priority.

Albania passed the Law on AIDS Prevention and Control in 2000. This legislation lays the legal foundation for prevention, treatment, and harm reduction interventions as well as anti-discrimination laws for PLWHA. To what degree the law is being implemented is unclear; one might infer from the financial sustainability problems of the health care sector

---

Table 13. Government Intervention and Institutional Arrangements—Albania

Testing	▓ According to legislation only state-owned institutions can offer HIV testing: 12 testing centers in Tirana and 12 prefecture blood centers, which are also responsible for routine blood screening
	▓ Testing is carried out only on voluntary basis, free of charge
	▓ Pre and post-test counseling are inadequate and poorly organized
Surveillance	▓ Statutory Major Disease-Based Surveillance System (MDBSS) monitors HIV/AIDS, but there is no population-based, nationally representative seroprevalence survey in the country
	▓ No systematic HIV sentinel surveillance undertaken among women attending antenatal clinics
	▓ Ministry of Defense was conducting HIV sentinel surveillance among recruits but funding threatened
HIV/AIDS Notification	▓ Data collected at the lowest level and sent through the District Epidemiological Services to the IPH
	▓ Includes clinical diagnosis but no information on CD4 count or viral load
	▓ Data considered inadequate in terms of quantity, quality and timeliness
Blood Safety	▓ Law on Blood Donation, Transfusion and Control of Blood Products passed in 1995 but remunerated blood donation continues
	▓ 7.1% of donated blood in 2001 was infected, out of which 1 case was HIV+
Prevention	Mostly carried out by NGO sector in TiranaPreventive activities include: condom promotion, peer education, safe sex promotion. Efforts are being made to integrate Life Skills and HIV/AIDS prevention education in school.
Treatment	▓ No adequate national guidelines for ART
	▓ The Tirana University Hospital Center (TUHC) treats patients
	▓ In 2004, about 50 adults with HIV infection were receiving ARV therapy

---

in general that funding to implement the law is highly inadequate. The Law on Prevention and Control of Infectious Diseases represented the first, and at the same time fundamental, constitutional law concerning infectious diseases. It requires mandatory notification and epidemiological measures for control and prevention. In addition, there are other laws that address specific areas of infectious disease control and health-related problems.

A National AIDS Program (NAP) has been established by the MOH within the Institute of Public Health (IPH). However, the NAP still does not have clear priorities regarding the targeting of preventive and harm reduction activities for vulnerable groups. National HIV/AIDS planning is hampered by inadequate surveillance; inadequate information on HIV prevalence and dynamics; high prevalence of risk behaviors; low levels of knowledge of HIV/AIDS; inadequate sexual and reproductive health education; inadequate information on sexual behavior, especially among young people; lack of/inadequate basic HIV/AIDS interventions; and lack of adequate funding.

Until recently, two people have only staffed the NAP, although the Government has recently allocated funds to enlarge its activities. The NAP has difficulty coordinating effectively with other government institutions and ministries because of rigid hierarchical and reporting structures. Albania has thus far focused its HIV/AIDS interventions on establishing a safe blood supply, and has started financing treatment with antiretroviral drugs for about 50 patients.

HIV/AIDS and STIs Surveillance

The statutory Major Disease-Based Surveillance System (MDBSS) of infectious diseases monitors 73 diseases that must be reported, including syphilis, gonorrhea, and HIV/AIDS. However, there has been no population-based, nationally representative serosurvey of HIV in the country. The Government has also funded a limited, Tirana-based HIV sentinel surveillance system, but its funding is precarious. Some seroepidemiological surveys have been carried out at different times among various sub-populations, including pregnant women, military personnel, health workers, persons going abroad for employment, and hospital patients. However, there is no systematic HIV sentinel surveillance undertaken among women attending antenatal clinics, a common (albeit imperfect) method of tracking HIV prevalence in the general population. Four sentinel groups are now being observed in Tirana to measure the trends of the epidemic: all pregnant women attending ANCs, new military recruits, women obtaining abortions at the Tirana Obstetric and Gynecology Hospital, and women with gynecological complications at the Tirana Obstetric and Gynecology Hospital. However, this sentinel surveillance system is now threatened by a lack of resources and political commitment (IOM and UNICEF 2002).

HIV/AIDS notification includes clinical diagnosis, but no information on CD4 count or viral load. Breakdowns of data are available by sex, age, residence, mode of exposure, and time of diagnosis. Surveillance of syphilis and gonorrhea has been achieved by clinician-based notification of clinically confirmed cases since the 1940s. Other STIs, including chlamydia, trichomoniasis, herpes virus infection, and human papilloma virus, are monitored through occasional cross-sectional surveys carried out by the Albanian Institute of Public Health. The data are sent from the lowest levels through District Epidemiological Services at a local level to the IPH at the national level. Though it is a good reporting system from an operational and functional point of view, the resulting data are considered inadequate in terms of quantity, quality, and timeliness.

Table 14. HIV Prevalence in Blood Donations, Albania 1996–2001

Year	Number of blood donations tested	Number of blood donations HIV+	Rate of blood donations infected
1996	18,692	1	5.3
1997	16,865	1	5.9
1998	16,131	1	6.2
1999	18,127	1	5.5
2000	15,200	0	0
2001	14,000	1	7.1

Source: European Center for the Epidemiological Monitoring of AIDS (2003).

The Institute of Public Health is recognized as the national reference laboratory and the expert lab for STI/HIV testing and diagnosis. Other specialized state laboratories are located at the University Hospital Center "Mother Theresa" in Tirana and in the 12 prefecture blood centers. The 12 blood centers are also responsible for routine screening of donated blood, and their laboratories serve as diagnostic centers for clients seeking testing on a voluntary basis.

Since 1993, all blood donations in Albania have been tested for HIV and Hepatitis B and C, with results reported to the federal level. In 1995, the Law On Blood Donation, Transfusion and Control of Blood Products was passed; it seeks to ensure the safety of the country's blood supply through obligatory blood screening and voluntary donations. However, remunerated blood donation continues, and the country is experiencing a blood donor crisis as it seeks voluntary donations.

The level of testing for HIV/AIDS and STIs is extremely low. Less than 0.7 percent of women are tested, and only 23 percent even know where to get tested. HIV testing is done by the ELISA test, with positive results confirmed by Western Blot at the IPH. There is limited capacity to test for syphilis with RPR, TPHA, FTA-Abs and ELISA. Testing patterns are not well understood, making interpretation of the notification data difficult. Private clinics carry out anonymous testing for STIs (mainly gonorrhea and syphilis).

According to the National Strategy on HIV/AIDS, HIV testing is carried out on a voluntary basis and is free of charge. According to current legislation, only state-owned institutions can offer testing for HIV. There are only three testing sites in Tirana: the Blood Bank, the IPH, and the University Hospital of Tirana. Outside Tirana, only blood banks in district centers can provide rapid tests for blood donors and volunteers. Confirmatory tests can only be carried out centrally, at the IPH or the University Hospital in Tirana. Specific problems related to HIV testing include the lack of regular and systematic reviews and evaluation of the HIV data from different groups, and different HIV testing methods (e.g. the Blood Bank in Tirana uses a different method than outlying districts). These problems bring into question the reliability and comparability of HIV data. Pre- and post-test counseling is only available at the IPH. Counseling is inadequate and poorly organized, despite some attempts to organize training based on WHO guidelines for medical staff at the key institutions and the involvement of some NGOs.

HIV/AIDS and STIs Prevention and Control in the Public System

The National Program for HIV/AIDS and STIs was established in 1993. The Program is led by the Institute of Public Health. Funds to support its work are derived from state budget contributions to IPH together with support from USAID, UNICEF, WHO, and other donors. In the mid-1990s, the old Soviet model of dermatovenerology dispensaries, which operated in Albania, disintegrated. These were gradually replaced by STI clinics set up in each of the 12 prefectures. However, over recent years their resource and funding base has experienced major decline, with a parallel decline in quality of diagnosis, treatment, and population coverage. STIs are mainly diagnosed on the basis of clinical features, although it is uncertain to what extent formal syndromic diagnostic approaches are used. Treatment of all STIs, with the exception of HIV/AIDS, is based on standard, official guidelines and carried out by gynecologists, dermatologists, and infectious disease specialists in both the public and private sector. USAID has organized an informal training for physicians (general practitioners) on syndromic management of STIs with a limited number of participants. UNFPA also provides training for GPs, but there is still a lack of adequate and routine training of GPs in this area.

Sexual education and issues related to HIV/AIDS are included in the school curricula to a certain level. A report prepared by MOH shows that 86 percent of parents and 95 percent of teachers are in favor of including sexual education in the school curriculum. Young Albanians say that they want to be better informed about reproductive health issues. This should take place in school as well as in the family. However, there are insufficient funds to support a serious level of health education at schools. Without improved education and prevention measures, and with a rising HIV incidence, young people will have a greater risk of infection. Access to family planning services and support is currently very limited. Less than half of Albanian women have ever had a gynecological examination, and only 23 percent of young women had ever heard of breast examination. Levels of awareness among rural women are much lower. Only 60 percent of women have any access to family planning services.

HIV/AIDS Treatment in the Public System

The 2000 law on HIV/AIDS provided an opportunity to include ARVs in the HIV/AIDS treatment package. In 2004, the budget included $150,000 for ARV, of which $112,000 had been spent by October. The MOH in cooperation with UNICEF purchased ARV drugs to treat 50 patients. Plans for 2005 are similar to 2004. The Department of Infectious Diseases at Tirana University Hospital Center (TUHC) "Mother Theresa" is the national center for treatment of HIV/AIDS and this department, together with the Dermatology Department of the same hospital, treats most cases of syphilis as well. Several physicians were trained to use ARV, and the IPH has been preparing national clinical guidelines and therapeutic protocols for HIV/AIDS andopportunistic infections.

HIV/AIDS Prevention and Control by NGOs

The limited drug abuse, HIV/AIDS, and STIs prevention activity in Albania is mainly carried out by NGOs. It is clear that the evolving NGO sector will provide future opportunities for HIV/AIDS prevention programs, however, like many other countries, most services are

---

Table 15. NGO Sector in Albania

- Soros Foundation: harm reduction project for Albanian NGOs
- Aksion Plus: harm reduction center for drug users in Tirana
- Cassa Emanuela: support to current and ex-drug users
- Asma-PSI: condom distribution
- Albanian Red Cross: peer education, HIV/AIDS prevention
- OSPES: awareness campaign
- Counseling Center for Women: hot line for cases of violence against women
- Terre des Hommes (Switzerland): prevention of trafficking of minors.

located in the capital city, Tirana. NGOs are a new phenomenon in Albanian society, one that has developed in the last ten years. Previously, such organizations were not allowed, and all activities were under the strict control of the Labor Party. Albanians participated in humanitarian activities through their local NGOs during the most difficult situations, especially during the Kosovo refugee crisis of 1999, when local NGOs succeeded in mobilizing more quickly than governmental bodies and the United Nations High Commissioner for Refugees (UNHCR).

Some of the NGOs and professional associations in the Albanian health sector are very large and well organized such as the Albanian Red Cross, an organization that has branches and volunteers in every district of the country. Others are more modest and operate in limited geographic areas. Most NGO financing originates from foreign bilateral and multilateral agencies. Many of the health sector NGOs are members of a large umbrella organization set up for the purpose of information exchange and coordination. Some specific NGO programs are listed below.

- Youth Networks such as Youth Parliament are doing Peer Education in school.
- Four NGOs (ASMA/PSI, NESMARK, JSI/TASC and AFPA) deal specifically with condom promotion, peer education, and health education.
- Several other NGOs such as Aksion Plus, Albanian Youth Council, and STOP AIDS, have been involved in peer education activities with a special focus on preventing HIV/AIDS and promoting safer sex.
- ALGA's main activities focus on HIV/AIDS prevention through grass-roots work focused in the distribution of condoms and lubricants to the gay community.
- SGA contributed to the changes in the legislation on homosexuality in 1995.
- Casa Dei Diritti Sociali is developing a project on harm reduction for Roma, and the staff works in close contact with minor Albanian male sex workers.
- CESVI is an organization implementing mainly projects focused on providing information at the community level.

Table 16. World Bank Support—Albania

Projects that address HIV directly	Projects that could include HIV/AIDS action	Analytical work that addresses HIV or risk factors
Albania Health Systems Development	▓ Trade and Transport Facilitation	Albania Poverty Assessment (non income-related dimensions of poverty)
▓ TA for development of HIV/AIDS strategy	▓ Social Sector Technical Assistance	
PRSC2	▓ Social Services Delivery	
▓ Improve financing of public health programs	▓ Education Reform	
▓ Develop HIV/AIDS Strategy		
PRSC3		
▓ Adoption and implementation of HIV/AIDS strategy, national education campaign		

▨ The NGO Medica Mondiale in Tirana comprises a multi-disciplinary team, which includes a gynecologist, psychiatrist, social worker, a nurse, and, among other activities, carries out group sessions that focus on personal hygiene, menopause, reproductive health, and family issues.

▨ The Albanian Family Planning Association, affiliated with International Planned Parenthood Federation since 1997, includes a program for training sex educators.

International Partner Organizations

External aid comes from foreign governments and international partner organizations. External aid accounts for a considerable proportion of Albanian general health care funding. During 1992 and 1993, it amounted to over one-third of the country's public health financing. The real value of foreign aid doubled in 1996, but since domestic spending on health also increased during this period, the foreign aid share of the total declined significantly in recent years. The main contributors have been the World Bank, the European Community Humanitarian Office (ECHO), the governments of Germany, Italy, France, Switzerland, Japan, Greece, and the United Kingdom, USAID, the Roman Catholic Church, OPEC Fund for International Development, UNICEF, UNFPA, and WHO. As in other countries in the region, international organizations such as the World Bank, UNDP, UNICEF, WHO, UNFPA, IOM and USAID provides support to the government efforts to combat HIV/AIDS.

The World Bank has been providing technical assistance for the development of the HIV/AIDS Strategy under the Albania Health Systems Project; and the Poverty Assessment tackled some of the drivers of the epidemic.

Table 17. International Support—Albania

UNAIDS TG	Organized a national conference on Policies of Prevention and Control of HIV/AIDS Epidemic in Albania
	Albania Program Accelaration Funds 2004–2005 approved
UNAIDS	The post of National Advisor was established in 1997, but in 2000 UNAIDS withdrew funding and the post no longer exists
UNFPA	Social marketing of condoms, youth-focused HIV/AIDS prevention, training health care providers on prevention
UNICEF	The Youth Parliament Project
	"Troc"—the national television youth news magazine
	Adolescent-focused peer education
	Reintegration of street children and trafficked children into schools
	Integration of basic Life Skills and HIV/AIDS education in the formal curricula of high school
	Establishment of Youth Friendly Health Services
	Support and facilitation to NGO network working in HIV/AIDS prevention
	Social campaigning in raising awareness among youth
	Support to the National Youth Strategy

(continued)

Table 17. International Support—Albania (*Continued*)

UNDP	Support to national planning and local NGOs for specific activities on HIV/STI prevention
UNDCP	Promoting healthy life-styles among youth
	Capacity building of the anti-drug police
	Prevention of drug abuse and trafficking
IOM	Policy level: Coordination of the National Strategy on Migration, support the development of HIV/AIDS national strategy targeting migrants and mobile groups.
	HIV/AIDS information, prevention and awareness raising
	HIV/AIDS Capacity building targeted at mass media, social workers and young TV stars
	Access to antiretroviral treatment: provided 2 years treatment to PLWHA
	Former Victims of Trafficking: Psyco-social, legal, medical, basic needs assistence, shelter, etc Reintegration assistance including vocational training and job placement.
	Prevention of trafficking: educational activities in schools and capacity building—regional.
	Assistance and reintegration of voluntary returned migrants
EUCARDS	Democracy and human rights
	Strengthening of public administration and judiciary
	Police and public order, customs, cross-border co-operation
	Statistics
	Development of infrastructure
	Local community development (including primary health)
	Agriculture, Environment, Education
ECHO	Financial assistance to health services rehabilitation
	ECHO concluded its operations in Albania in 2002
CIDA	Southern Europe HIV/AIDS Prevention: aims to develop national and regional responses to HIV/AIDS. Focuses on youth prevention.
	Child Rights
	Local Initiatives Program
	Humanitarian Assistance to Extremely Vulnerable Refugees
	Assistance to Refugees and Host Families
	Relief Supplies to Kosovar Refugees in Albania
	Supported Axsion Plus Harm Reduction Center in Tirana
USAID	Health Sector Improvement: works to improve access, use and quality of key health services, primarily those used by women and children. Activities include reforming primary health care system's management structure; encouraging the Ministry of Health to incorporate family planning and reproductive health services in proposed changes; and fighting HIV/AIDS.
PSI	Social marketing project promoting and providing condoms

CHAPTER 7

Profile: Bosnia and Herzegovina

Table 18. Epidemiology—Bosnia and Herzegovina

Population Population Reference Bureau	3.9 million
Registered HIV cases Federal IPH 2004	Bosnia and Herzegovina: 101
HIV/AIDS Prevalence UNAIDS 2003	<0.1
New HIV Cases Federal IPH 2004	Bosnia and Herzegovina- 9
Modes of Transmission Federal IPH 2004	▓ IDU 14% ▓ Heterosexual 54% ▓ MSM 15% ▓ Blood 3% ▓ Unknown 14%
Registered STIs cases Federal IPH, RS IPH	Syphilis 　2003—25 　2002—25 　2001—50 Gonorrhea 　1987—557 　Since 1998 <50 annually

(*continued*)

Table 18. Epidemiology—Bosnia and Herzegovina (*Continued*)

TB notification rate 2004 Federal IPH, RS IPH	63 per 100,000
Vulnerable Groups World Bank 2003 UNICEF 2002	Youth
	▓ Median age of population 35.1
	▓ Mean age when first used drugs 15.4
	IDU
	▓ Estimated number 6,000–10,000
	▓ 70% share needles
	▓ 50% tested for HIV
	▓ 37% positive for Hepatitis C
	▓ 62% do not consider drug use to be risk factor
	CSW
	▓ Estimated number 11,000–15,000
	▓ 65 % use drugs
	▓ 35% sometimes or never use condoms
	▓ 84% understand that they have increased risk
	▓ 98% have been tested for HIV
	MSM
	▓ Highly stigmatized and discriminated
	▓ 77% use drugs,
	▓ 10% tested for HIV

Epidemiological Overview

HIV/AIDS

From 1985 to end of 2004, there were 101 HIV cases officially reported in Bosnia and Herzegovina, of which 44 had already developed AIDS and died; the status of 33 notified cases is unknown. According to data from the Institute of Public Health, of the 101 reported HIV infections by the end of 2004, at least 54 percent were transmitted heterosexually, 15 percent) via MSM, 14 percent via IDU, and none through mother-to-child transmission. According to data released by EuroHIV (2003), no HIV infections had been detected among blood donations screened for HIV antibodies from 2000 through 2002. The highest incidence is among the age groups 25–29 and 40–44 years old.

According to IHP data, there has been a cumulative total of 44 AIDS-related deaths among the 55 AIDS cases reported through the end of 2004. The first AIDS case was registered in 1986 and the first HIV case in 1989 (IOM and UNICEF 2002). From 1986 to 1991, the AIDS prevalence per 100,000 was 0.25 (11 cases), and from 1992 to the end of 2004, AIDS prevalence was 1.2 per 100,000. Approximately 90 percent of AIDS cases were men. More than half of the infections were transmitted through sexual contact. According to the data submitted by the cantonal/regional levels of the Institute of Public Health, 28 percent of all AIDS cases are

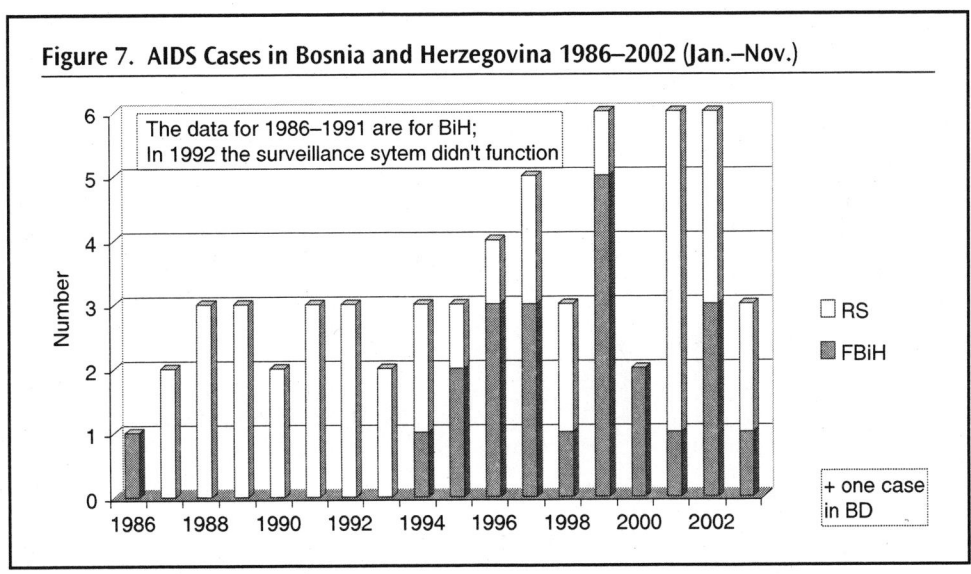

Figure 7. AIDS Cases in Bosnia and Herzegovina 1986–2002 (Jan.–Nov.)

The data for 1986–1991 are for BiH;
In 1992 the surveillance sytem didn't function

□ RS
▨ FBiH

+ one case
in BD

Source: Federal IPH, RS IPH.

among heterosexual people, 24 percent among MSM, and 24 percent among IDUs. About 8 percent were identified on blood and blood products, and the mode of transmission was unknown in 16 percent of the cases (Bosnia and Herzegovina AIDS Commission 2003).

Sexually-transmitted Infections

Due to weak public health infrastructure, both syphilis and gonorrhea are severely under-reported in Bosnia and Herzegovina. Fifty cases of syphilis were reported in 1987, but only four in 1991. Since 1998, the annual incidence of syphilis was more than 10 cases per year. Patients with active STI are not routinely tested for HIV, and there is no information on

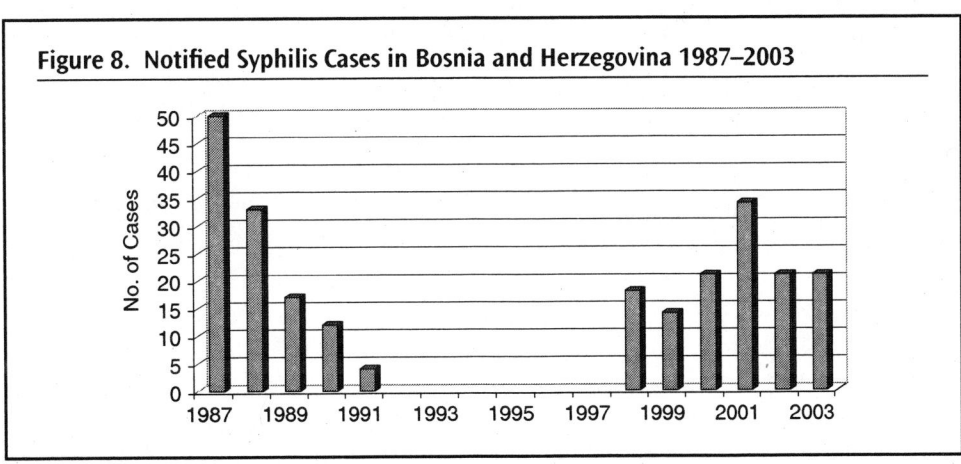

Figure 8. Notified Syphilis Cases in Bosnia and Herzegovina 1987–2003

Source: Federal IPH, RS IPH.

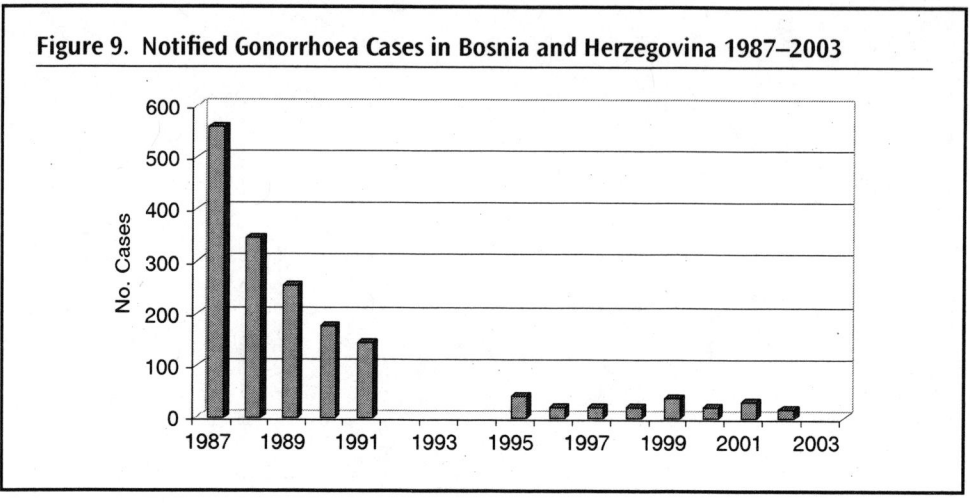

Figure 9. Notified Gonorrhoea Cases in Bosnia and Herzegovina 1987–2003

Source: Federal IPH, RS IPH

the level of STIs or HIV and modes of transmission in high-risk groups. The decline in annual notifications does not reflect the true trends of syphilis incidence within the territories. In 2003, the reported notification rate was 0.54 per 100,000 population. This extremely low rate almost certainly reflects a significant breakdown in either access to clinical services, shifts in source of care, or changes in health care provider's willingness to report cases.

Since 1998, the number of notifications of gonorrhea cases in the Federation has been less than 50 cases a year, and except for an outbreak in 2000, it has been decreasing ever since. In 1987, in pre-war Bosnia and Herzegovina, 557 cases of gonorrhea were reported. No breakdown by sex or age was available. Again, the decline in annual notifications does not reflect the true trends of gonorrhea incidence within the territories. Although chlamydia is a notifiable disease, no cases have been reported. It is very unlikely that this reflects the true situation. A recent two-year study has shown that among 120 women in two clinics in Sarajevo, 8 tested positive on chlamydia trachomatis (Mahmutovic and others 2003).

Vulnerability to HIV/AIDS: Contextual Factors

According to the Population Reference Bureau, Bosnia and Herzegovina's mid-2003 population was 3.9 million people (PRB 2003), whereas the UN Population Division put the 2003 population at 4.2 million. Bosnia and Herzegovina's annual population growth rate in 1995–2000 was 3 percent, but this figure is projected to fall to 0.07 percent during 2010–2015 (UN 2003). Bosnjaks account for 48 percent of the population, followed by Bosnian Serbs (34 percent) and Bosnian Croats (15.4 percent). Approximately 40 percent of Bosnia and Herzegovina's population is Muslim, followed by Christian Orthodox (31 percent), Catholic (15 percent), and Protestant (4 percent) (U.S. Department of State 2003c).

About 19 percent of the population is under age 15 (PRB 2003), and the median age in 2000 was 35.1 (UN 2003). Given the declining rate in the natural increase of population, increasing life expectancy, and emigration of the youth, the population of Bosnia and Herzegovina is aging (Bosnia and Herzegovina Council of Ministers 2003). In 2001, Bosnia and Herzegovina's Human Development Index (HDI)[8] was 0.777, ranking 66th out of 175 countries (Wong 2002).

In 1992, Bosnia and Herzegovina declared independence from the Socialist Federal Republic of Yugoslavia (World Bank 2003b). The war (1992–1995) caused widespread physical damage. Over 10 percent of the pre-war 4.4 million population was killed or wounded and over half of the population was internally displaced or refugees abroad (Bosnia and Herzegovina Council of Ministers 2003). Two-thirds of homes were damaged, with one-fifth totally destroyed. Between 170,000 and 240,000 persons were wounded. Of these, 100,000 were severely wounded and 25,000 left with permanent disabilities. It is estimated that at least 16,000 children died and that perhaps another 40,000 were wounded (Cain and Jakubowski 2002). An estimated 30–40 percent of hospitals were destroyed and 30 percent of health care professionals were lost to death or emigration.

In early 1996, a peacekeeping force of 60,000 NATO-led Implementation Force (IFOR) troops from over 30 countries took up positions around the country. IFOR was the forerunner to the current NATO-led Stabilization Force (SFOR) that is still stationed in Bosnia and Herzegovina. Following three years of civil war, the Dayton Accord was negotiated in November 1995. Dayton acknowledged the bitter ethnic divides that had let to war by establishing a government structure with a weak central State. It also provided for a strong international policy and military presence and an international overseer—the Office of the High Representative (OHR). In the context of this agreement, the Priority Reconstruction Program was also designed and endorsed by Bosnia and Herzegovina authorities and international donors; the program had an overall budget of over US$5.1 billion (Cain and Jakubowski 2002).

In November 2003, the EU approved a feasibility study assessing the readiness of Bosnia and Herzegovina for European integration. Bosnia and Herzegovina must make significant progress in a number of areas identified as priorities for action, including more effective public administration, post-accession criteria for democracy and human rights, tackling organized crime, managing asylum and migration, and developing reliable statistics (EU 2003).

Economy

With the exception of Macedonia, Bosnia and Herzegovina was the poorest republic in the Socialist Federal Republic of Yugoslavia. Bosnia and Herzegovina is a lower-middle-income country with gross national income (GNI) per capita of US$1,540. Approximately 56 percent

---

8. The Human Development Index (HDI) incorporates average life expectancy at birth, adult literacy and combined primary, secondary, and tertiary gross enrollment ratios, and gross national per capita income. An HDI of 0.800 or above = high human development; 0.500–0.799 = medium human development; less than 0.500 = low human development.

Table 19. Vulnerability Factors in Bosnia and Herzegovina

GNI per Capita World Bank 2003	US$ 1,540
Unemployment Government 2002	38.7%
Poverty World Bank 2003	20%
Mobility	▦ >250,000 IDPs in Bosnia and Herzegovina ▦ >240,000 IDP in RS ▦ 23,500 in Brcko District
Trafficking	▦ Bosnia and Herzegovina is destination as well route of trafficking to Western Europe ▦ 25% women working in bars and night clubs are victims of trafficking

of GDP is created in the services sector, 29 percent in industry, and 14 percent in agriculture (World Bank 2003). Bosnia and Herzegovina's Council of Ministers (2003) estimates that with the loss of GDP from 1992 to date, the overall financial impact of the war amounts to over US$100 billion. By the end of the war in 1995, economic production had contracted by over 90 percent, physical capital was extensively destroyed, and GDP fell by 80 percent. In 1996, a major donor assistance program set the stage for reconstruction and economic recovery, and 60 multi- and bilateral donors committed nearly US$1.9 billion to the effort. Whereas recovery, spurred by reconstruction, began in 1996 in Bosnia and Herzegovina, donor assistance and recovery began later in the entity of Republika Srpska (RS) because of the effect of international sanctions.

The combination of large-scale donor assistance, sound economic policies, and the initiation of structural reforms have yielded good results in reconstruction and economic recovery. Since the end of the war in 1995, the country has made extraordinary progress in addressing many of its post-conflict challenges. Average annual GDP growth in the post-war period reached 25 percent, much of its infrastructure was restored, and an increasingly functional administration established. However, serious challenges remain. The country remains highly dependent on aid, and prospects for the emergence of a self-sustaining economy is delayed to the latter part of this decade (World Bank 2002a).

Unemployment (coupled with inactivity or exclusion from the labor force) is a major problem for Bosnia and Herzegovina and it inhibits post-war recovery and the transition to a market economy. In 2002, there were over 400,000 unemployed persons in Bosnia and Herzegovina, yielding an official unemployment rate of 41 percent in a population age group that is economically active. At the end of 2002, women represented 46 percent of the overall number of unemployed. Bosnia and Herzegovina's Poverty Reduction Strategy Paper (PRSP) states that the rate of women's participation in the labor force is the lowest of any country in Southeastern Europe. All registered unemployed persons have the right to health care, and their contributions are paid from the entity budgets (Bosnia and Hersegovina Council of Ministers 2003).

Poverty

According to the Bank's 2003 Poverty Assessment, some 20 percent of the population still lives below the poverty line, with an additional 30 percent highly vulnerable to poverty. Moreover, serious distortions in the social safety net adversely affect the poor and threaten the financial sustainability of the system. The education level is the single most significant factor affecting the risk of poverty in Bosnia and Herzegovina. About 60 percent of the poor live in households in which the head of the family has only primary or less education. The probability of a household falling below the poverty line is almost tripled in this situation. There is some relation between the ethnic structure and levels of household income. In Croat-majority areas, 7 percent of households are poor based on income levels. In Bosnjak-majority areas, this percentage ranges from 22 to 25 percent, and in Serb-majority areas, between 40 and 43 percent. Over half of ethnic minority households in RS are poor, and in the Croat-majority areas of Bosnia and Herzegovina 16 percent of ethnic minority households are poor. In Bosnjak-majority areas, about 25 percent of ethnic minority households are poor (Bosnia and Hersegovina Council of Ministers 2003).

Altogether, the unemployed, displaced persons, the disabled, and members of families of soldiers killed during the war account for less than half of the poor in Bosnia and Herzegovina. About 63 percent of the poor live in households (families with children), in which at least one person is employed; less than 20 percent of the poor live in households in which the head of the family is not working. In mid-2003, there were about 260,000 beneficiaries of social welfare in Bosnia and Herzegovina—about 7 percent of the population of Bosnia and Herzegovina and of RS. Additionally, 125,000 beneficiaries were registered for child-care programs.

The Government has approved a Poverty Reduction Strategy Paper prepared with technical support from the Bank, UNDP, multi- and bilateral external assistance and in cooperation with civil society. Bosnia and Herzegovina's PRSP of November 2003 briefly mentions HIV/AIDS in its analysis of health sector priorities. However, HIV/AIDS is not specifically mentioned in the PRSP's Action Plan. Among the actions included in the plan are: passage of the Law on Public Protection from Infectious Diseases, and creation of a new public health strategy where society would become responsible for the health of the individual and the community, and would use various inter-sectoral activities to create changes in individual behavior and improvements to health (World Bank 2004a).

Mobility

Bosnia and Herzegovina has a highly mobile population, including refugees, IDPs, returnees, rural-urban migrants, labor migrants, transport workers, international workers, military personnel, victims of trafficking, sex workers and Roma (IOM and UNICEF 2002). Mobility often entails regroupings of family units and exposure to new sexual networks, which may have significant ramifications for HIV transmission. According to May 2003 data from Bosnia and Herzegovina's Council of Ministers, there are currently 281,652 displaced persons residing in Bosnia and Herzegovina (35 percent from the territory of Bosnia and Herzegovina and 65 percent from RS); 243,386 displaced persons in RS; and about 23,500 in Brcko District. Over 300,000 Bosnians live abroad; of whom about 50 percent have no clear status.

Vulnerable Groups

The country has experienced major conflicts and upheavals and, inevitably, there are substantial levels of commercial sex work, injecting drug use, and displacement. However, there are no plausible estimates of the numbers of injecting drug users or commercial sex workers.

Youth. In 2003, there were 606,000 students in Bosnia and Herzegovina (World Bank 2004a). Overall, women are slightly less likely than men to be literate (91 vs. 98 percent). The long-term departure of young and educated people from Bosnia and Herzegovina is a significant drain on human capital. Over 92,000 young people left the country in the first five years following the war due to unemployment, the economic crisis, inability to afford adequate housing, and political instability. Almost two-thirds of young persons indicate that they are ready to emigrate given the opportunity. Unemployment is likely the major problem affecting youth in both urban and rural areas.

A Rapid Assessment among school-aged drug users was carried out in 2001–2002, in Sarajevo, Tuzla, Mostar, Banjaluka and Brcko, with support of UNICEF, WHO and OSI (Baran 2002). This sample of young people reported many factors that led them towards drug and sex risk behavior, including high levels of social and economic stress and unemployment, poor education, family dissatisfaction with level of education and social status, family problems, conflict and instability, lack of attention, abuse, alcoholism, and lack of adequate leisure activities. Marijuana and ecstasy were reported as easy to obtain. The average age of first sexual intercourse was reported as 16.5 years for males and 17.4 years for females. On average, males reported four lifetime sexual partners and females one. The majority of young people reported that they did not use condoms, and significant numbers believe condoms are primarily of value for contraception, not for prevention of STIs and HIV.

International Workers and Peacekeepers. In 2002, there were an estimated 40,000 international workers (including NATO and UN peacekeepers) in Bosnia and Herzegovina (DFID 2002). By December 2003, SFOR started the reduction of troop levels from about 12,000 to a deterrent force of around 7,000 (NATO 2003).

Sex Workers and Trafficking. Although prostitution is illegal in Bosnia and Herzegovina, both commercial sex work and trafficking are pervasive. Similar to other countries in the region, it is difficult to provide reliable figures on commercial sex work, but NGOs and IOM estimate that there are 11,000–15,000 CSW in Bosnia. In late 2002, Human Rights Watch reported that from 1992 through 1995, thousands of women and girls suffered sexual violence, including abuse in camps and detention centers scattered throughout the country. There was significant trafficking of women and girls for forced prostitution, including approximately 25 percent of the women and girls working in nightclubs and bars. Since 2000, the Government has become more involved in organizing a systemic approach to combat trafficking. The UN Convention Against Transnational Organized Crime and the Anti-trafficking Declaration of SEE were signed and a Working Group on Trafficking was established to coordinate activities among the Government, international organizations, and NGOs. A National Plan of Action was also developed and was approved by the Council of Ministers in December 2001. However, the problem still persists.

Organized crime, creating corruption and trafficking in drugs and humans, continues in the post-war period, with routes from Albania, Kosovo, and Montenegro through Bosnia and Croatia. Effective border surveillance is difficult due both to the large, uncontrolled number of tracks and border crossing points between the RS and Montenegro, and to the corruption within local police and the State Border Service (UN Security Countil 2003). With the breakup of the former Yugoslavia, porous borders, along with massive socio-economic challenges, have given criminal networks fertile ground to traffic in human beings for the growing sex industry. This region is increasingly used by traffickers, both as a destination and as a major route to Western Europe. The first reports of human trafficking in Bosnia and Herzegovina were issued by NGOs and IPTF in 1998 (IOM and UNICEF 2002), and note that trafficking occurs mostly from Moldova, Romania, and Ukraine and, to a lesser extent, Russia, Belarus, Kazakhstan, and Serbia and Montenegro. Although the presence of international civilian and military personnel has contributed to the trafficking problem in Bosnia and Herzegovina, the local criminal situation sustains it (U.S. Department of States 2003b).

MSM. There is little information available on MSM in Bosnia and Herzegovina. However, similar to other countries of the region, same sex interaction is highly stigmatized and the MSM community remains largely underground. Among homosexual men interviewed by the Rapid Assessment in Tuzla, there was a strong feeling that they were highly stigmatized. The mean age of MSM interviewed by the RAR was 21 years; 77 percent used drugs; all had had sexual intercourse; but only 70 percent thought that they were at risk of HIV or other STIs. Only 10 percent had been tested for HIV. Of those who used drugs, 96 percent had sex under the influence of drugs. The mean age at first sexual intercourse was 17 years; 47 percent had between two and five sexual partners in the past year; only 7 percent always used condoms during sex; and 27 percent had sex in return for money or drugs (Wong 2002a).

Drug Users. There is a growing problem with intravenous drug use, as in other countries in the region. It is estimated that there are at least 6,000–10,000 IDUs in Bosnia and Herzegovina. During the last several years, the age of new IDUs has been getting lower, affecting children as young as 13 and 14 years of age. Among drug users interviewed by UNICEF's RAR, the majority started using drugs between 16 and 19 years of age. There is a predominance of males among drug injectors. Alcohol, marijuana, and ecstasy are the most popular drugs, and heroin was the main drug used by those injecting. About 70 percent of injectors reported sharing needles and syringes. The majority of drug users reported frequent sexual activity while under the influence of drugs. Around 70 percent of IDU thought that that they were not at risk of getting HIV/AIDS, while 62 percent did not feel their drug use to be a problem. Among IDUs, 97 percent reported having sexual intercourse, and 50 percent had been tested for HIV. Of sexually active IDUs, 70 percent sometimes or never used condoms during sex, and 9 percent had sex in return for money or drugs. According to internal reports of the Federation MOH, 37 percent of tested IDUs were positive for Hepatitis C, which indicates the practice of sharing needles. Needle sharing is actually considered among IDUs as a symbol of "brotherhood." In the UNICEF RAR study, IDUs reported that existing treatment conditions on the psychiatric wards are inadequate. Many stated that they would accept methadone or community treatment (Wong 2002a).

Roma. A highly marginalized minority group in Bosnia and Herzegovina is the Roma population. Estimates of the total population range from 17,000 to 80,000, making them the largest ethnic minority. Although many have integrated into communities, many are still mobile. They have been subject to constant displacement during the war and constant discrimination. A low illiteracy rate of 23 percent and low attendance rates at primary schools have resulted in an almost total absence of high school, vocational, and university education. Many have no identification papers so, consequently, they cannot qualify for general social security programs and specially adapted programs (Bosnia and Herzegovina Council of Ministers 2003).

HIV/AIDS Awareness and Knowledge

Stigma associated with HIV/AIDS may be high. In the 2000 Multiple Indicator Cluster Surveys in Bosnia and Herzegovina and FR Yugoslavia (excluding Kosovo), 24 percent of women in Bosnia and Herzegovina agreed with at least one of two discriminatory statements about people living with HIV/AIDS (Bernd and McKee 2003). The UNICEF MISC 2000 found that among women ages 15–49 years, 97 percent had heard of HIV/AIDS, and almost half of them knew all three-transmission modes. Half believed that having only one uninfected sex partner could prevent HIV transmission. Half believed that using a condom every time one had sexual intercourse could prevent HIV/AIDS transmission, and 39 percent agreed that abstaining from sexual intercourse prevents HIV transmission (IPH 2002). Differences across age groups were not particularly large; the percentage of women who knew the two HIV avoidance methods (sticking to one uninfected partner and using condoms), ranged from 47 percent among ages 20–24 to 35 percent among ages 45–49. The level of education was important: 25 percent of women with primary or no education knew three ways to avoid HIV, compared to 51 percent of women with secondary or higher education. Seven in ten women ages 15–49 correctly believed that a healthy looking person can be infected with HIV/AIDS. Among 15–19 years old, this figure was 72 percent. Seven in ten women in Bosnia and Herzegovina knew that HIV/AIDS can be transmitted from mother to child. When asked specifically about the mechanisms through which mother to child transmission occurs, 68 percent stated that transmission during pregnancy was possible, 59 percent that transmission at delivery was possible, and 54 percent agreed that HIV can be transmitted through breast milk.

Table 20. Knowledge, Attitudes, and Practices in Bosnia and Herzegovina

KAP	37% IDUs positive for Hepatitis C
RAR 2002	70% IDU share needles
	70% thought that that they were not at risk of getting HIV/AIDS
	77% MSM use drugs
	96% MSM had sex under the influence of drugs
	24% of women agreed with at least one of two discriminatory statements about people living with HIV/AIDS

Governance

After the war, a central state government and two autonomous entities were established: the Federation of Bosnia and Herzegovina (FBiH) and the Republika Srpska (RS); and one district, District of Brčko (DB). Each entity has its own parliament, government, military forces and police, as well as education, health care, and other public services. FBiH is divided into 10 cantons, each with its own government and assembly (Wong 2002a). The establishment of a heavy administrative public sector apparatus for a country the size of Bosnia and Herzegovina contributed to rapidly growing public expenditures. The massive unemployment further aggravated this pattern, with the public sector assuming the role of employer of last resort. Absence of financial and non-financial incentives for the staff in key government institutions is further weakening the capacity of those institutions to change. Qualified staff is usually seeking employment with international organizations or abroad. Premature decentralization, as a result of peace agreements, seriously affected the efficiency of the public institutions in Bosnia and Herzegovina. The key institutions, unready for change, have largely continued to function in the same manner as prior to the war, while the administrative structure and governing framework have changed dramatically. At the same time, newly created institutions lack the capacity to operate effectively.

War eroded the integrity of public institutions and the rule of law, allowing widespread corruption (Cain and Jakubowski 2002). According to Transparency International's Corruption Perceptions Index 2003, Bosnia and Herzegovina ranked as the 64th-most corrupt country in the world out of 133 countries surveyed. The PRSP (Bosnia and Herzegovina Council of Ministers 2003) notes that corruption affects the poor:

> ... especially hard, whether it is related to visiting a doctor, acquiring rights to some form of social assistance, obtaining documents, education, return of property or employment, because they often have no other way to ensure the necessary services. Displaced persons, the rural population, children and young people are often forced to pay for such services because they are not properly accepted or recognized by their communities, and lack the channels of communication that could enable them to demand their rights.

Bosnia and Herzegovina's PRSP notes significant human rights violations in Bosnia and Herzegovina, primarily affecting minority ethnic groups, displaced persons and returnees by being unable to exercise rights to free and equitable enjoyment of their property, to acquire an education, to enjoy access to health care or social services or to participate in the labor market. This may result in weakened social organization and decline in authority of Government and institutions. Increased crime rates, accidents and disease create a sense of insecurity and increase in the incidence of poverty among all categories of the population. Education, health care, and social protections are falling below human rights standards.

Health Care in Bosnia and Herzegovina

While the infrastructure was restored relatively rapidly after the war, the basic organization of the health care delivery system has not changed significantly. In FBiH, the health system administration is decentralized, with each of the 10 cantonal administrations having responsibility for the provision of primary and secondary health care through their own Ministry of Health. In RS, authority over the health system is centralized, with planning, regulation, and management functions held by the Ministry of Health and Social Welfare in Banja Luka. Compared to other social sectors, ongoing reform of the health sector is both broader and in a more advanced stage. Yet deeper reforms are needed to ensure the sustainability of the system and overcome prevailing weaknesses in efficiency, equity, and quality of health services.

Within the health system, overall, there is insufficient attention to public health, health promotion, and prevention. The curriculum in Family Medicine supported by CIDA Canada and the Bank attempts to redress this problem. The Bank, with co-financing from the Italian Government, has supported the strengthening of primary health care through the introduction of family medicine in pilot cantons/regions in both Entities. Acceptance of the family medicine model has grown rapidly well beyond pilot sites and surveys report improved patient and provider satisfaction with the system. In addition, referrals are decreasing (Cain and Jakubowski 2002). A recent completed evaluation of the implementation of the project and specifically of family medicine interventions shows that the efforts were highly successful. The Bank is working with both Ministries of Health to prepare a new project—Health Scale-up Project to expand the effective implementation of family medicine nation wide. The project is scheduled for approval in 2005.

Health legislation in both Entities allows for private providers. To date, private provision of care is almost exclusively limited to specialist outpatient services. Health insurance does not cover provision by the private sector. Household data show, however, that over 10 percent of people who sought outpatient services utilized private providers. Beyond the Bosnalijek factory and small-scale production in pharmacies and hospitals, most drugs are imported. Pharmaceutical supply during the war and postwar period (1992–2000) was primarily channeled through humanitarian aid programs, covering up to 70 percent of supplies. In a large number of cases, this scenario heavily influenced the choice of therapy, which often depended more on the type and quantity of drugs available rather than local needs. An Institute for Quality Control of Medicines (IQCM) has now been established in both Entities. The current fragmented system drains scarce public resources at the expense of necessary health care services, forcing pharmaceutical prices to rise because of low purchasing volumes. This affects procurement of drugs and equipment, in particular, as well as secondary and tertiary services. In 1998, WHO studied the pricing of specific drugs inside Bosnia and Herzegovina and found that the best local offer was more than double that obtained on the international market (Cain and Jakubowski 2002).

Funding of Health Services

According to NHA, public expenditure on health care in 2000 was nearly 8 percent of GDP, whereas private health care expenditure represented almost 5 percent of GDP (UNDP 2003). According to Bosnia and Herzegovina's PRSP, taking into consideration informal out-of-pocket payments for health care services, brings total health care spending (public and private) to about 13 percent of GDP, which is very high for a lower-middle-income country such as Bosnia and Herzegovina. About 37 percent of health care spending is on primary health care, 35 percent on secondary care, and 18 percent percent on tertiary care. Currently, there are no direct HIV/AIDS-related allocations in the national budget.

In the FBiH, 17 percent of the population does not have health insurance; and 35 percent of the population in the RS does not have health insurance. There are large differences in insurance coverage between the poor and non-poor populations. In RS, close to 50 percent of the poor are uninsured, while in the Federation 30 percent of the poor are not insured. Utilization of health services by insured and uninsured varies greatly, although payments do not, suggesting problems with access and equity in a system that is supposed to assure universal coverage. The groups more strongly affected by the low insurance coverage are the unemployed and those out of the formal labor market. Health insurance does not provide protection even for those who have insurance, in case of serious illness, whereas the uninsured are particularly at risk. Given the high costs of health care, this scenario can further push households into poverty.

Health services for young people are free up until the age of 14 years. After the age of 15, young people have to pay a participation fee for services received (about 30 percent of the total price). It appears that many young people are not covered by health insurance, though exact data is not available. This applies particularly to marginalized young people such as injecting drug users, sex workers, and young women who have been trafficked. There are inequalities in service provision based on area of residence and social status. Young people from rural areas, refugees, and internally displaced young people are among the most disadvantaged. Further, there is very low health insurance coverage for people living in rural areas.

Government and Civil Society action on HIV/AIDS

Strategic, Policy, and Regulatory Framework

In 2002, Bosnia and Herzegovina adopted the UN proposals to fight AIDS. Soon afterwards, the Bosnia and Herzegovina AIDS National Advisory Board was established. The Council of Ministers adopted the National Strategy for Prevention and Fighting Against AIDS in February 2004. The National Advisory Board is leading the efforts to implement the Strategy. Since 2003, there is a network of cantonal HIV/AIDS coordinators in the Federation. The FBiH coordination operates under the Federation Ministry of Health, while the RS coordination is under the RS Ministry of Health and Social Welfare (IOM and UNICEP 2002; UNAIDS 2001b). The Bosnia and Herzegovina Council of Ministers has appointed the Ministry for Civil Afairs, along with UNAIDS technical support, as coordinator for all activities related to the operations of the National Advisory Board for Action against HIV/AIDS. Members of NAB are representatives from the entity governments, including representatives from the Brcko District, NGOs, and international agencies.

In 1999, the Sarajevo Canton MOH and FBiH Government adopted a Program of Primary Prevention of Drug Addiction. In addition, a policy document for a Federation Program of Alcoholism and Drug and Substance Abuse has also been drafted (Wong 2002a). In 2002, the Bosnia and Herzegovina NAB developed the National Strategy for Prevention

Table 21. Government Intervention and Institutional Arrangements in Bosnia and Herzegovina

Intersectoral coordination	▪ Council of Ministers established the National HIV/AIDS Committee, which includes NGOs and international organizations
National HIV/AIDS Strategy and Legislation	▪ National Plan for Action to combat trafficking approved in December 2001
	▪ Strategy for Prevention and Fighting Against HIV/AIDS 2003–2008 was developed by the National Advisory Board for Action against HIV/AIDS and approved in February 2004
Government institution responsible for HIV/AIDS	▪ Ministry for Civil Afairs chairs National Advisory Board for Action against HIV/AIDS
	▪ Institute of Public Health collects and analysis epidemiological data on HIV/AIDS

and Fight Against AIDS (2003–2008) in preparation for an application to the Global Fund to Fight AIDs, TB, and Malaria. In 2004, the National Strategy was published with UNICEF support, with five main golas:

▪ Prevent transmission and spread of HIV.
▪ Ensure adequate treatment, care, and support to persons living with HIV/AIDS (PLWHA).
▪ Create a legal framework for the protection of ethical principles and human rights of PLWHA.
▪ Assure coordination and sustainable capacity development in the fight against HIV/AIDS.
▪ Encourage and strengthen links with international institutions in the fight against HIV/AIDS.

The local office of UNHCHR has joined the UN Theme Group on HIV/AIDS to examine strategic ways to review the legal frameworks while incorporating a human rights approach (IOM and UNICEF 2002). Since 1987, AIDS has been a notifiable disease under the Law on Protection of the Population from Communicable Diseases. According to UNICEF, however, this law does not conform to the principles of the Convention on Human Rights (Wong 2002a). Since December 2001, both FBiH and RS have been considering implementing mandatory HIV testing for high-risk groups. There are numerous human rights issues surrounding this plan, and human rights advocacy groups contest the implementation of such a program. There is also a law under consideration that would require a mandatory seven-year prison sentence if a person with HIV knowingly infects another through sexual intercourse. UNHCHR is contesting the language of the proposed law.

The Government realizes the significance of the continuous cooperation between the governmental and non-governmental sectors, multisectoral cooperation, and the need for a multidisciplinary approach in the fight against HIV/AIDS. Although the efforts of the Ministries and public health authorities to combat HIV/AIDS are commendable, at the policy level, the capacity of the multiple health ministries to set strategic goals, formulate policy options, and implement them remains limited. The Government recognizes that additional work has to be carried out to take into account gender dimensions and human rights; to increase intersectoral cooperation, and to disseminate and use available data. However, since the approval of the National AIDS Strategy, the following has been accomplished:

- A mechanism for prevention and treatment of HIV and AIDS was established. The network of National Coordinators (NC) on HIV/AIDS was set up (18 NCs in total: 10 in the Federation, 7 in the RS, 1 in the Brcko District).
- VCCT Centers were set up and cooperation with NGOs in dealing with HIV/AIDS in the country was developed in the same locations as NCs. Operating Protocols for VCCT Centers are under discussion.
- Several UN agencies and NGOs are involved—UNFPA YFHS for sexual and reproductive health 4 centres (Bihac, Banja Luka, Mostar and Brcko); UNICEF EVYP 2 centres (Zenica and Tuzla); Project Hope is training health professionals and NGOs; XY established NGO APOHA (PLWHA) and is dealing with people living with HIV/AIDS.
- The roles and responsibilities of the CCM were readdressed, and a monitoring and evaluation (M&E) system is being developed. A sub-regional Workshop on M&E was attended by the National Group representatives. The follow-up National Workshop on M&E was held in October and the M&E Action Plan was designed. The basic national program indicators have been agreed at the workshop.
- CRIS (UNAIDS Country Response Information System) data processing and analysis were discussed and one pilot location (Tuzla) was selected for CRIS implementation.
- Establishing reporting on VCT coverage from the network of local PHIs. Reported data will be entered in CRIS.
- Three studies will be undertaken to identify the HIV/AIDS status of drug users, MSM and CSW, as well as their access to the services.
- A HIV/AIDS surveillance system for drug users is being established, which should enable monitoring trends of risk behaviors among IDUs.

HIV/AIDS and STIs Surveillance

An integrated system of routine surveillance of communicable diseases does not exist at the national level; rather, each entity has its own data collection, based on physician reports. The Canadian Public Health Association has carried out a Rapid Assessment of the Bosnia and Herzegovina HIV/AIDS and STI surveillance system. A joint reporting for both entities for EuroHIV was also recently established.

Separate epidemiology departments and Institutes of Public Health throughout the country are in charge of the surveillance of communicable diseases in their specific area, including the surveillance of HIV/AIDS and STIs. These are under the national supervision of the Federation Institute of Public Health in the FBiH and the Institute of Public Health in RS. All communicable diseases are reported by physicians to the cantonal/regional IPHs using a preprinted report form, which is similar for the entire country.

The forms are then sent to the IPH at the entity level (Federation IPH in FBiH and the IPH in RS). The notification period for routine diseases is one week in FBiH. The notification period in RS and DB is on a monthly basis, while in the case of a suspected outbreak it is one to two days.

The numerous reporting systems currently in place reflect the vestiges of the older surveillance system of the former Yugoslavia, which do not reflect modern public health disease control and prevention needs. Reporting of HIV diagnoses and the notification of such infections has been severely disrupted over recent years. Moreover, data on HIV/AIDS in FBiH were found to be inconsistent across the sources. This is partly caused by population displacements during the 1990s and the subsequent division of the country. During the 1992–1995 war, HIV testing equipment was unavailable, and since then the public health infrastructure has remained weak. However, significant efforts are being made to improve the notification system.

Notifications of syphilis may be relatively complete however. Physicians consider syphilis a serious illness and therefore report it more seriously than other STIs. Gynecologists are not reporting gonorrhea, reasons for which are unclear, so gonorrhea is severely underreported. Very few cases of chlamydia have been reported, which is explained by the outdated lab equipment, insufficient number of trained personnel, and lack of financial resources for the new equipment, training, and reagents.

Despite the availability of tests, testing rates are among the lowest in Europe. ELISA testing is offered in both Entities (FBiH and RS). Testing for HIV-1/2 includes serological testing, that is, two ELISA tests, Western Blot, and PCR, in line with WHO recommendations.

Table 22. Government Intervention and Institutional Arrangements in Bosnia and Herzegovina

Testing	Testing rate is among the lowest in Europe
	ELISA testing is available in several centers in FBiH, RS and DB
	Voluntary testing is now free of charge
	No pretest counseling is available, posttest counseling is done in several centers
	Positive samples are sent to central laboratories in Sarajevo and Belgrade for Western blot
Surveillance	Integrated system of routine surveillance not available
	Data from cantonal level is collected by Federal Institute of Public Health of BiHa and IPF of Republika Sprska (RS)
HIV/AIDS Notification	Notification is done at cantonal levels using preprinted report form
Blood Safety	Free testing for HIV is offered to all blood donors
Prevention	Mostly carried out by NGO sector
Treatment	Four Clinics of Infectious disease in Bosnia and Herzegovina and one in RS offer treatment
	ARV are included on the essential drugs list
	Drug therapy is not covered by statewide medical insurance
	No universal or systemic guidelines for ART

Voluntary testing is available in VCTT Centers (11 so far), all transfusion centers and for blood donors in both FBiH and RS. Sites include: Institute for Transfusion Medicine in Sarajevo; Central Microbiological Laboratory at Koševo Hospital; RS Institute of Public Health; and Clinic for Infectious Diseases (CID) Immunology Laboratory, in Banja Luka. In the event of a positive test using ELISA methodology, the blood samples are sent to the Clinical Center in Sarajevo for confirmation using the Western Blot test. ELISA positive samples in RS are sent to Belgrade for confirmation using the Western Blot test. HIV tests for blood donors are free of charge (IOM and UNICEF 2002). Since 2005, voluntary, anonymous and confidential testing for HIV/AIDS is free of charge in the Federation, and it is planned to make free testing available in RS and DB.

In FBiH and RS, HIV testing is officially confidential, according to an International Organization for Migration coding system. However, in the event of a positive ELISA, the blood sample and full name of the patient were forwarded for further analysis. The Federation Ministry of Health (MOH) has been developing a system for HIV testing in an attempt to ensure voluntary access and full confidentiality. However, the Federation still faces lack of laboratory capacity for diagnosis of HIV infections.

There is no systematic pretest HIV counseling available in either entity. Reportedly, post-test counseling is available at two locations within FBiH (the CIDs in Sarajevo and Tuzla), and at one site in RS (CID in Banja Luka). However, there are no mental health professionals on site at these facilities. Post-test counseling, if any, occurs when a doctor or patient specifically calls a mental health professional from the outside, if anyone is available. There are no special services in Bosnia and Herzegovina for psychological counseling of patients with HIV/AIDS. PLWHA are sometimes referred to a psychiatrist, if one is available (IOM and UNICEF 2002).

HIV/AIDS, STIs, and Drug Use Prevention and Control in the Public System

There are no systematic strategies to improve HIV/AIDS awareness and harm reduction programs (HR) for highly vulnerable groups. The Government does not provide any harm reduction or needle exchange programs, and there are very limited services provided by the NGO sector. Bosnia and Herzegovina law prohibits possession of any quantities and form of illegal drugs, and providing a safe room for injecting can be prosecuted and tried for criminal offense. Despite the undefined legislation, the National Advisory Board has identified the need to establish harm reduction programs in Bosnia and Herzegovina under the AIDS Strategy.

The Institute of Mother and Child Health Care (Belgrade, Serbia) trained six health care providers and 30 young people (peer educators) from five different towns in RS in 2002 in counselling services for young people. This training preceded the establishment of Young People's Counselling Centers, which were attached to primary health care centers (PHCs) in the five towns where peer educators were trained. Funds will be required for equipment and possible renovation in three of the centers. Training health care providers and young people is expected to continue until the whole of RS is covered.

A joint project in FBiH, between the Ministry of Education, Science, Culture and Sports and the MOH, was initiated in May 2000, entitled "Healthy Lifestyle in Schools." Its purpose is to promote healthy lifestyles and increase awareness of HIV/AIDS prevention in primary schools. In FBiH, the three medical faculties, the Bank, and local government cooperated to provide peer education and life skills education to 100 schools in 10 cantons; the project is expected to reach 10,000 students across FBiH (IOM and UNICEF 2002).

HIV/AIDS, STIs, and Drug Use Treatment

In mid-2003, UNAIDS (2003b) published data indicating that 10 percent of adults in Bosnia and Herzegovina with advanced HIV infection were receiving antiretroviral therapy (ART). Universal and systematic hospital guidelines or protocols for ART are beeing developed for the management of HIV/AIDS patients, but have not yet been officialy adopted by MOH. HIV/AIDS patients are referred to four clinics in Sarajevo, Tuzla, Mostar and Banja Luka. Although all these clinics report that they offer both in- and out-patient services, the quality of these services is reported to be poor. Treatment consists of limited antiretroviral therapy. Yet, facilities for determining CD4 cell counts and measuring viral load are only available at the CID in Sarajevo and HAART treatment is also available only in Sarajevo and Tuzla. Since September 2003, treatment is available in the Bosnia and Herzegovina clinics with funding from Federal Solidarity. ARV drugs are included in the essential drugs list, and ART is now available although problems with importation of drugs persist.

Doctors working with PLWHA are trained in Croatia, Italy, and France and then organize peer education in Bosnia and Herzegovina. There appears to be limited awareness of treatment of HIV/AIDS cases among health professionals outside the CIDs. In some cases, health professionals may be reluctant to treat PLWHA due to lack of training or discriminatory attitudes. Furthermore, hospitals and clinics do not always have the proper protective equipment, such as gloves, masks, and post exposure preventive kits, to reduce the risk of exposure for health workers.

There are no specialized clinics for diagnosis, treatment, and management of STIs in Bosnia and Herzegovina. Thus, patients with STIs are largely treated in outpatient clinics in primary health centers and in general hospitals across the country. General physicians may refer patients to specialists, depending on the patient's symptoms. If genital infection is suspected, patients are referred to gynecologists and urologists, and if clinical symptoms include skin changes, they are referred to dermatologists. HIV/AIDS patients are referred to infectious disease specialists. It is likely that the majority of patients are treated syndromically due to the limited availability of STI tests. There is emerging evidence of the use of private sector services by young people (in particular, pharmacists for treatment of STIs and gynecologists for abortions), as well as self-medication for certain conditions (Homans 2003).

Medical treatment for drug withdrawal for IDUs is currently only available at the University Clinic in Sarajevo. Although a methadone replacement program is available, no clinical protocol and therapeutic guidance has been developed, and it is reported that quality of treatment is poor and inefficient. Some individuals go abroad for treatment, which is very expensive and an available solution for only a few.

HIV/AIDS Prevention and Control by NGOs

During the last several years, many local and international NGOs have been supporting efforts to prevent HIV and support PLWHA. Cooperation and networking among NGOs have been established. The concern is that the NGO sector is highly dependent on donor funding, thereby impeding the sustainability of its interventions, and there is inadequate

---

Table 23. NGO Sector in Bosnia and Herzegovina

- Youth Against AIDS Action (YAAA), Sarajevo, has been identified as one of the most efficient local groups for HIV/AIDS education and prevention.
- Campaigns take place in numerous areas of Bosnia and Herzegovina, including organizing and distributing brochures in relevant languages to CSWs and trafficked women (UNAIDS 2001).
- With UNICEF, supported a survey of young people's knowledge.
- Began peer education activities in October 2000.

---

support from the public and the government. Interventions are also made difficult in other ways. For example, NGOs disseminate harm reduction information and sterile needles to IDUs. However, under current legislation, needle exchange programs are difficult to implement in a systematic manner.

Many local NGOs are supported by international organizations and NGOs, as described below:

- *IOM* is finalizing a project for HIV/AIDS prevention in Mobile Populations across SEE. IOM has cooperated with many local and international NGOs, several local and national Government entities, and other groups to assist women, especially women who have been involved in trafficking. With UNFPA and funding from CIDA, IOM provides reproductive health information, referrals for trafficked women to gynecological and counseling services in Bosnia and Herzegovina. IOM also tries to ensure women have access to this support upon return to their home countries.

- *CESVI* (Cooperation and Development Agency) is an Italian NGO funded by the Italian Ministry of Foreign Affairs. The HIV/AIDS project runs through 2004, and concerns young people and all aspects of their education. Phase I of CESVI provides medical equipment for the laboratory in the Banja Luka General Hospital to improve the testing facilities for HIV/AIDS. Phase II focuses on the establishment of a network that will involve all youth organizations in Bosnia and Herzegovina that support PLWHA. Workshops will include various campaigns and distribution of materials related to HIV/AIDS. Phase II will involve CESVI and four other Italian NGOs.

- *Italian League for Fight Against AIDS-Center for Human Rights and Public Health* (LILA-CEDIUS), implemented with IOM a preparatory counseling course for general practitioners in Banja Luka, as well as seminars on the prevention of HIV infection and drug use for youth football team trainers in Sarajevo.

- *NBV*, a Swedish NGO, supports anti-drug campaigns within schools and among teachers.

- Through *RiskNet,* funded by USAID, Population Services International (PSI) supports NGOs engaging in prevention activities, including referrals to treatment centers; VCT; and distribution of condoms, clean needles (not funded by USAID), and educational materials. This cross-border project covers Bosnia and Herzegovina, as well as Macedonia, Romania, Croatia, and Bulgaria (Open Society Institute 2003).

▨ *Open Society Fund* in Bosnia and Herzegovina (OSF–BH) is committed to the development of an economically and socially sustainable country marked by good governance and an open, democratic civil society. The Fund's programs focus on local governance, education, women, Roma, youth, networking, and student enterprises (UNAIDS 2003c).

▨ *IFRC and the Red Cross Society of Bosnia and Herzegovina* (RCS) donated testing materials to the transfusion centers until the beginning of 2000. IFRC and RCS are implementing peer education and lifestyle programs throughout Bosnia and Herzegovina. Contraception, prevention of STIs with special emphasis on HIV/ AIDS, and gender violence are the main activities of this program. A nationwide network of Red Cross Peer Educators has been developed in 2000–2001. Information booklets on Safe and Sound Sexuality, HIV/AIDS and STIs, designed for young people, are available in all municipal Red Cross organizations throughout the country.

▨ *CARE International* is supporting peer education programs in selected schools.

International Partner Organizations

Although there are a large number of international agencies present in Bosnia and Herzegovina, HIV/AIDS has not yet been addressed in a systematic or coordinated fashion. However, HIV/AIDS is included in the Action Plan for Health within the Stability Pact framework that is being prepared by the WHO Regional Office for Europe, together with other partners. The following agencies are active in the prevention and control of HIV/AIDS:

▨ *UNICEF* supports activities through local NGOs, including life skills and peer education, voluntary counseling and testing, and research on young people who sell sex. Together with WHO, UNICEF has initiated support to the State Strategic Planning process in Bosnia and Herzegovina, and both Health Ministries have indicated their interest in starting to prepare a situation and response analysis and a multisectoral HIV/AIDS prevention strategy in Bosnia and Herzegovina. UNICEF

Table 24. World Bank Support in Bosnia and Herzegovina

Projects that address HIV directly	Projects that could include HIV/AIDS action	Analytical work that addresses HIV or risk factors
Basic Health Project	*SITAP*	
Public health strengthening component, including health promotion activities supported through health innovation grants which addressed HIV/AIDS.	▨ Access to basic services and sector governance *Essential Health Services* ▨ Hospitals infrastructure rehabilitation *Health Scale-up Project (FY05)* ▨ Expand family medicine model and health promotion activities at PHC Trade and Transport Facilitation	

Table 25. International Support in Bosnia and Herzegovina

UN Theme Group	▓ First established in Bosnia and Herzegovina in 1997 and lasted until 1998. It was reestablished in March 2001
	▓ Technical working groups of local experts and NGO representatives have been established in both Entities
UNAIDS	▓ Between 2002 and 2003, UNAIDS involved in training-of-trainers programs to build the HIV/AIDS-education capacity of Bosnia and Herzegovina military and police forces
UNFPA	▓ Funding reproductive health education through peer counseling at national level
	▓ Preparation of policy papers on reproductive health.
	▓ Supports peer education work of Youth Action against AIDS
	▓ Development of model of youth-friendly centers to be implemented under the GFATM grant
UNODC	▓ Currently supporting a harm reduction program with the Forum of Solidarity in Tuzla
UNICEF	▓ Supports activities through local NGOs including life skills and peer education, harm reduction and counseling
	▓ With Ministry of Education and Pediatric Association established "Educating School Children in the Prevention of Sexually-transmitted Diseases and HIV/AIDS"
	▓ Supports a pilot project on life skills
	▓ Together with the Open Society Institute (OSI) supported a survey of young people's knowledge of HIV/AIDS in Bosnia and Herzegovina
UNMIBH	▓ Supported the Epidemiological Surveillance working group
UNHCR	▓ Monitors and responds to human rights concerns, as well as supports gender mainstreaming and gender analysis
WHO	▓ Support to the State Strategic Planning process in Bosnia and Herzegovina
	▓ HIV/AIDS surveillance system
	▓ Reporting on HIV/AIDS from both entities to EuroHIV
	▓ HIV preventive interventions
	▓ Blood safety
CIDA/CPHA	▓ Southern Europe HIV/AIDS Prevention/Child Rights: 2001–2004: project aims to develop national and regional responses to HIV/AIDS. It focuses on youth prevention and increases socio-medical success for children with special needs.

conducted the RAR. Together with OSI, UNICEF has also supported a survey of young people's knowledge about HIV/AIDS in Bosnia and Herzegovina. UNICEF, with financial support from CIDA and technical assistance provided through the Canadian Public Health Association, is implementing HIV prevention activities through government and non-government sectors.

▓ *UNFPA* is funding reproductive health education through peer counseling at a national level, implemented by the Red Cross Society of Bosnia and Herzegovina.

The International Federation of the Red Cross (IFRC) is the executing agency for this project. UNPFA has also supported the preparation of policy papers on reproductive health. In partnership with UNICEF and UNESCO, UNFPA supported the first national peer education workshop in Bosnia and Herzegovina, which brought together youth NGOs from across the country. UNFPA is working closely with IOM to support programs related to trafficked persons. UNFPA has developed a model for youth-friendly services, which would be implemented under the GFATM grant.

- The *Canadian Public Health Association*, through a regional public health project in the Balkans region funded by CIDA, has provided financial support and technical assistance to strengthen local responses to HIV/AIDS through contributing to the development of the HIV/AIDS strategic planning process, and most recently, in carrying out a rapid assessment of the HIV/AIDS and STI surveillance system.
- *Project Hope* have also provided support to HIV/AIDS prevention activities.

The *World Bank* has supported health promotion activities and has financed Public Health Innovation Grants, including for HIV/AIDS control through the Basic Health Project. It will also support health innovation grants through the Health Scale up Project.

CHAPTER 8

Profile: Macedonia

Table 26. Epidemiology—Macedonia

Population	2.1 million
Registered HIV cases MoH 2004	69
HIV/AIDS Prevalence UNAIDS 2003	>0.1
New HIV Cases MoH 2004	1998—3s
	1999—5
	2000—3
	2001—3
	2002—5
	2004—6
Modes of Transmission MoH 2004	▓ 65% heterosexual
	▓ 14% MSM
	▓ 11% IDU
	▓ 5% MTCT
Registered STIs cases IPH	▓ Syphilis—17
	▓ Gonorrhea—144
	▓ Chlamydia—38
	▓ STI Men/women ration: 7.5/1

(continued)

Table 26. Epidemiology—Macedonia (*Continued*)

TB notification rate	▓ 32 per 100,000; 648 reported cases
World Bank 2001	▓ High rates of TB in prisons (143 per 100,000) and among refugees (109 per 100,000)
Vulnerable Groups	Youth
UNICEF 2002	▓ 45% under 30 unemployed
	▓ Mean age IDUs 21; when first injected drugs 17
	▓ 75% of infected between 20–39 years
	IDU
	▓ Between 12,000–15,000 IDUs
	CSW
	▓ Between 5,000–6,000 foreign CSW
	Prisoners
	▓ 1,500 prisoners (98% male)
	Juvenile Delinquents
	▓ Mean age 17
	▓ 39% IDUs
	▓ 74% had sexual intercourse
	▓ 24% tested for HIV
	Mobile Population
	▓ 25% of Macedonians go abroad as seasonal workers

Epidemiological Overview: HIV/AIDS and STIS

HIV/AIDS

The true epidemiological picture for HIV/AIDS in Macedonia is not clear although the overall reported incidence of HIV/AIDS is low. There is a relatively weak national surveillance system that lacks specific data for the most vulnerable groups in society. From 1987 to the end of 2004, only 69 people had been found to be HIV positive in the country. These figures are too low for any relevant conclusions on the predominant mode of transition. The first HIV infection was registered in 1987, and the first AIDS case in 1989. According to the MoH, of the 69 reported HIV infections, 65 percent) were transmitted heterosexually, 14 percent) were diagnosed in MSM, 11 percent in IDUs, and 5 percent through mother-to-child transmission (MTCT). According to the Macedonia National Multisectoral HIV/AIDS Commission (2003), the first reported HIV infection and AIDS case were both hemophiliacs infected via tainted, imported blood products. In 2003, EuroHIV did not provide data on transmission via unsafe blood/blood products.

Figure 10 presents AIDS notifications and deaths between 1989 and 2001. By the end of 2004, 18 people were known to be living with HIV, and 46 had died. Most cases of HIV/AIDS are among men (69 percent), and in the age groups 20–29 and 30–39 years of age. The ratio of men to women was 2.4:1 among AIDS cases and 2:1 among HIV cases.

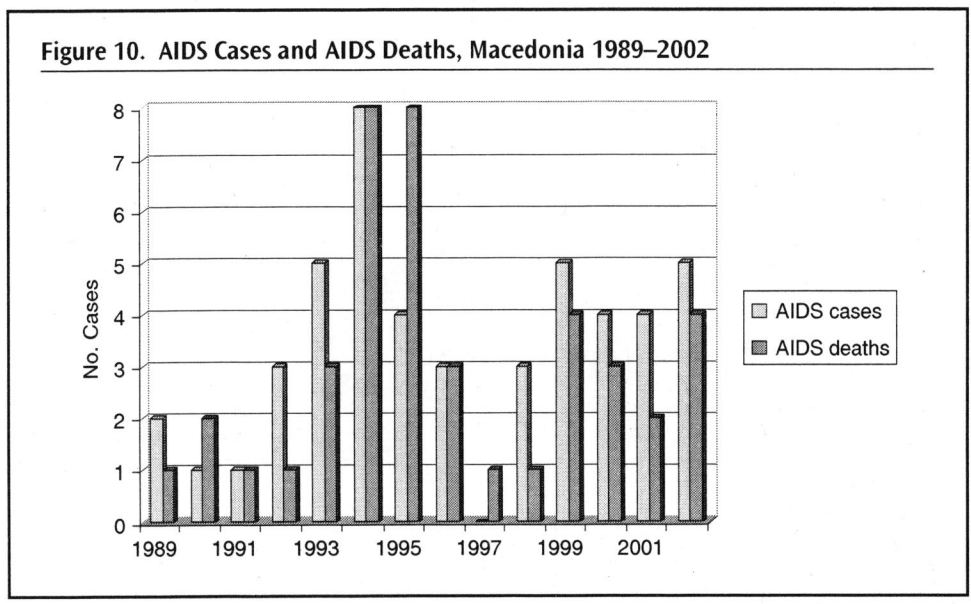

Figure 10. AIDS Cases and AIDS Deaths, Macedonia 1989–2002

Source: IPH Macedonia.

According to the *Macedonia HIV/AIDS National Strategy 2003-2006*, which provided data for 46 AIDS cases, 8.7 percent were hemophiliacs; no data for the separate category of transfusion were provided.

Sexually-transmitted Infections

Gonorrhea and syphilis have been recorded in Macedonia since 1980. Data from 1995 to 2002 are shown in Figures 11 and 12. Figure 11 shows the number of notified cases of

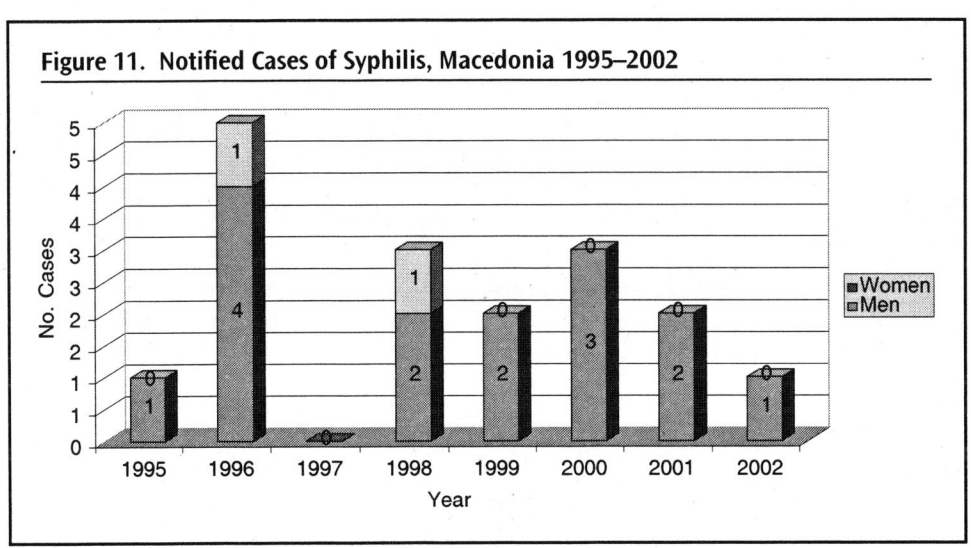

Figure 11. Notified Cases of Syphilis, Macedonia 1995–2002

Source: IPH Macedonia.

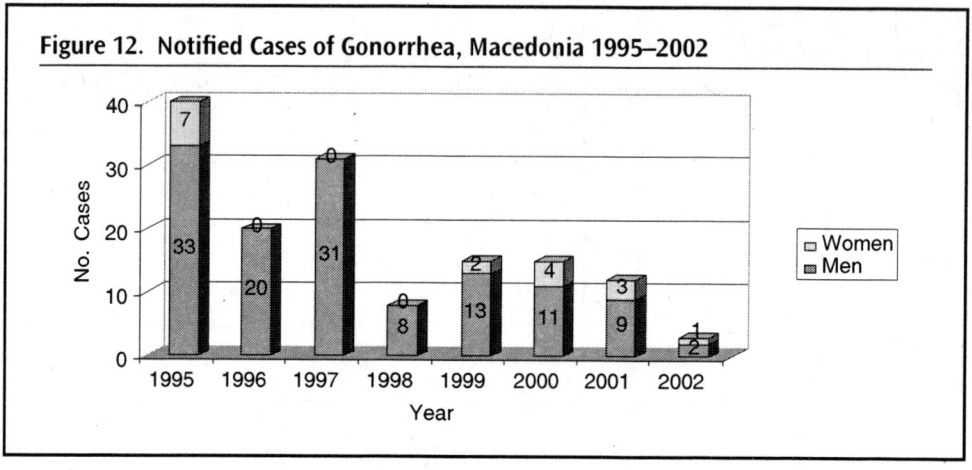

Figure 12. Notified Cases of Gonorrhea, Macedonia 1995–2002

Source: IPH Macedonia.

syphilis in the country between 1995 and 2002. During 1995–2002, a total of 17 syphilis cases were reported. In 2002, the notification rate per 100,000 population was less than 0.05. This seems impossibly low as a realistic measure of incidence within this population and certainly points to very significant surveillance deficiencies. Most cases (two-thirds of the total) were among men aged 20–39 years. Between 1995 and 2002, a total of 144 cases of gonorrhea were notified, again with the most affected group being men aged 20–39 years (two-thirds of all cases). The ratio of men to women was 7.5:1. Again these numbers seem impossibly low as a realistic measure of incidence within this population. During the 1999–2002 period, 38 cases of chlamydia were reported—14 cases in 1999 and 2001 and 5 in 2000 and 2002.

Vulnerability to HIV/AIDS: Contextual Factors

The United Nations officially refers to Macedonia by its provisional name, The Former Yugoslav Republic of Macedonia, pending the outcome of UN-mediated negotiations between Macedonia and Greece. The country's mid-2003 population was 2.1 million people. Macedonians account for about 64 percent of the population, followed by ethnic Albanians (25 percent), Turks (4 percent), Roma (3 percent), and Serbs (2 percent). Approximately 65 percent of Macedonia's population is Eastern Orthodox Christian, followed by Muslim (29 percent) and Catholic (4 percent) (U.S. Department of State 2003d). Approximately 22 percent of the population is under age 15 (PRB 2003) and the median age is 33 (UN 2003).

Macedonia declared independence from the Socialist Federal Republic of Yugoslavia (SFRY) in late 1991. The new Macedonian Constitution took effect in November 1991, and called for a system of government based on a parliamentary democracy. Macedonia was the only republic of former Yugoslavia whose secession in 1991 did not spur ethnic or other armed conflict. However, by late 2000, many ethnic Albanians questioned their minority

Table 27. Vulnerability Factors—Macedonia	
GNI per Capita World Bank 2001	US$1,690
Unemployment World Bank 2003	36.7%
Poverty Household Survey	▓ 20% ▓ >75% poor with less than primary education
Mobility	▓ 25% of labor force seasonal workers abroad ▓ No HIV/AIDS interventions targeted to the mobile population
Trafficking	▓ No quantitative data available on trafficking victims ▓ Country is destination for, and a major route to Western Europe for trafficked victims

protection and demanded participation in the government (U.S. Department of State 2003d). In early 2001, fighting erupted between Macedonian government forces and ethnic Albanian rebels in the northwest region of the country. This led to some 40,000–50,000 citizens seeking asylum abroad and significant levels of internal displacement. In August 2001, an internationally mediated ceasefire led to the disarmament of insurgents, overseen by NATO, a presidential amnesty for most combatants, and a peace agreement signed by the leaders of the major political parties. By 2003, violence had subsided in the conflict-affected areas, most displaced persons had returned home, and the police had established an active presence in most communities.

Although Macedonia escaped hostilities within its borders until 2001, tensions were often high throughout the 1990s because of the spillover effects of nearby conflicts. During the same period, the intermittent closing of borders to the north and the south isolated Macedonia geographically and impeded international trade. In 1999, the Kosovo conflict pushed about 350,000 refugees across the border into Macedonia (the equivalent of 17 percent of the country's population). The crisis severely strained internal stability and economic management within Macedonia, severing key trade and transport links to the north and presenting a considerable humanitarian challenge in managing and caring for Kosovar refugees. With the military intervention and financial assistance of the international community, there was an early end to hostilities, most refugees quickly returned home, and the Macedonian economy rapidly recovered. However, the unresolved final status of Kosovo remains a potential flashpoint for ethnic tensions and continues to constrain the regional economic and political outlook.

Economy

The first half of the 1990s saw a marked decrease in living standards in Macedonia. Over the last few years, the inflation rate and GDP have stabilized, but unemployment figures have steadily increased. Since the late 1960s, Macedonia has had high rates of unemployment, which have worsened with the transition to a market economy. Currently, about

45 percent of the Macedonian workforce is employed in industry and commerce, followed by 31 percent in services, and 24 percent in agriculture (U.S. Department of State 2003d).

According to the World Bank, Macedonia's economy had been contracting for over six years at the time of independence in 1991. By 1996, however, inflation fell to single digits and the fiscal deficit to 1.4 percent of GDP. Over the next several years, the pace of economic growth increased, price stability was preserved, and fiscal balance was largely achieved. However, the 1999 Kosovo crisis resulted in a double-digit rate of decline of industrial production and a severe deterioration of the fiscal balance. The 2001 civil conflict further disrupted economic momentum. Although direct conflict damage was limited, output fell by 4.5 percent. In 2001, Macedonia's GNI per capita was US$1,690, ranking it 111 out of 208 countries. GDP growth during 2000–2001 was –4.1 percent. Privatization, although rapid, has generally favored insiders, which has significantly restricted post-privatization restructuring (World Bank 2003d). In 2002, the recovery of the economy was slower than expected.

While FYR Macedonia's economy has undergone dramatic changes since 1990, there appears to have been relatively little adjustment in public administration employment levels. Aggregate employment in the non-economic sphere declined only slightly in the 1990s. The resulting skill deficit in critical areas adversely affects the capacity of FYR Macedonia's policy-making institutions, as they are less able to effectively support Government and Parliament in adjusting policies to evolving economic and social realities. Political divisions within and among key institutions (particularly after the internal conflict in 2001), and fragmentation and ill-defined functions and roles among key institutions further weaken the capacity to formulate and implement policies and key public health functions of the state.

Poverty

Extreme poverty affects one-quarter of Macedonia's population. Data from the 2000 Household Budget Survey indicate that 20 percent of the population falls below the national poverty line (about US$75 per month in 1996 prices). Macedonia's Interim Poverty Reduction Strategy Paper (2000 PRSP) notes that poverty is the result of two factors: fall in aggregate consumption during the 1990s; and rise in inequality in its distribution. Two-thirds of poor households live in rural areas. Most of the households have multiple members and low educational status; they are socially more isolated, with a higher mortality rate. According to the Government, some of the worst-off rural households are the elderly, with only social assistance benefits or a small pension as income. There is a strong correlation between the level of education and poverty. Although education levels in Macedonia are reasonably high, over 75 percent of the poor have only some primary school education. High-risk groups, whose members are unlikely to achieve a satisfactory level of education, include rural children, Muslims (especially females), Roma, and those with special physical or psychological needs. Macedonia's 2000 Interim PRSP does not mention HIV/AIDS.

Mobility

In 1999, Macedonia temporarily hosted about 360,000 Kosovar Albanians and other refugees fleeing the violence in Kosovo. The refugee influx put significant stress on Macedonia's weak social infrastructure. Following the resolution of the conflict, the overwhelming majority of refugees returned to Kosovo (U.S Department of State 2003d; UNICEF 2003b). The 2001 conflict within Macedonia led to 80,000 IDPs and 50,000 Macedonians seeking asylum in other countries. An estimated 25 percent of Macedonians live abroad, many of whom are seasonal laborers who return periodically to Macedonia. As yet, however, no HIV/AIDS interventions specifically target mobile populations (Macedonia National Multisectoral HIV/AIDS Commission 2003). Given the high mobility trend that characterizes the socio-geographic functioning of the Republic of Macedonia, there is an urgent need for responses that address the mobile groups, particularly in relation to vulnerability to HIV/AIDS.

Vulnerable Groups

Although the official number of people living with HIV/AIDS is very low, and data about vulnerable groups is scant, the information about epidemic drivers such as poverty, mobility and commercial sex work; knowledge and practices of vulnerable groups and lack of preventive activities is a cause for concern.

Youth. About 45 percent of the unemployed are under age 30 (Macedonia National Multisectoral HIV/AIDS Commission 2003). According to a recently conducted survey, the vast majority of the Macedonian youth plan to move abroad in the future. UNICEF's RAR[9] found that young people engage in risky sexual behavior and many do not always use condoms. They often have more than one partner and have sex while under the influence of one or more substances. Among youth who are reported not to use drugs, 19.4 percent percent had had sexual intercourse. Of these, 62 percent thought that they were at risk of HIV or other STIs, and 5 percent had been tested for HIV. Further, of those who had sexual intercourse, 40 percent had between two and five sexual partners in the past year; 60 percent always used condoms during sex; and 8 percent had sex in return for money or drugs. Among youth in institutional care, 10 percent had used drugs, 43 percent had sexual intercourse; 66 percent thought that they were at risk of HIV or other STIs; and 5 percent had been tested for HIV.

The military service recruits 18 to 27 year-old males for 10-month enrollments in Military School and Academy. Participants must pass several medical tests, including syphilis, and Hepatitis B and C. The HIV test, however, is not mandatory. The recruits are only tested for HIV if there is a medical indication that they may be infected. No pre- and post-HIV test counseling is offered. Each class of new recruits receives one lecture about STIs.

International Forces. Prior to the 1999 NATO bombing campaign in Yugoslavia, the number of NATO troops in Macedonia peaked at 17,000. Macedonia now hosts about 150 NATO troops who support NATO operations in Kosovo and assist Macedonia's efforts to

---

9. UNICEF's Rapid Assessment and Response on HIV/AIDS Among Especially Vulnerable Young People in South Eastern Europe (RAR). Field work for the Macedonia RAR, funded by CIDA, was undertaken from August 2001 to March 2002. A questionnaire was administered to 1,755 young people in Skopje, Kumanovo, Strumica, Prilep, and Ohrid, including those in secondary school, aged 14 to 19 years; IDUs, aged 10 to 24 years; young MSM or bisexuals (includes female bisexuals); youth in institutional care, aged 10 to 18 years; and youth in correctional institutions, aged 10 to 18 years.

reform its military to meet NATO standards (U.S. Department of State 2003d). Little is known about the impact of the international troops on the general Macedonian population. KFOR troops from Kosovo take "rest and recuperation" in Macedonia, and there are reports that they use brothels and bars, particularly in the tourist areas (IOM and UNICEF 2002). Previously (from 1992–1998), the UN Preventive Deployment Force (UNPREDEP) in Macedonia patrolled the borders with Serbia and Albania.

Sex Workers and Trafficking. There are no accurate figures for the number of sex workers in Macedonia. However, IOM reported that Macedonia has moved from being a transition country for human trafficking to a recipient country and to a country of origin for commercial sex workers (CSW). Estimates show that there are still 5,000–6,000 foreign CSW in the country. The National Multisectoral HIV/AIDS Commission (2003) also confirms that the socio-economic crisis has led to an increase in sex work. The commission reports that sex workers often lack primary education and health insurance and face discrimination and violence. There are other indications that this part of the region is increasingly being used by traffickers, both as a destination and as a major route to Western Europe. Specifically, Macedonia is a country of transit and destination for women and children trafficked for prostitution from the former Soviet Union and Eastern Europe, notably Ukraine, Moldova, Romania, and Bulgaria. Some victims remain in Macedonia, whereas others are trafficked to Albania, Kosovo, or Italy.

According to the U.S. State Department, the Government of Macedonia fully complies with the minimum standards for the elimination of trafficking. The Government has shown increasingly effective law enforcement activities in ethnic Albanian areas not under Government control during the 2001 conflict, and in areas where trafficking activity is prevalent. Given that it is a post-conflict country with limited resources, the U.S. Department of State (2003c) does note, however, that the low conviction rate relative to arrests is an area of concern, as is the integrity of some members of the judiciary.

MSM. Participants in UNICEF's RAR stated that casual sex was fairly common among MSM. Awareness about condoms and how to use them was low. Participants reported that drug use only included alcohol and cannabis (Wong 2002a). The RAR indicates that 30 percent of MSM interviewed had had 5 to 12 sexual partners in the course of the year, and 21 percent said that they have had 3 to 7 one-night stands. A large degree of risk is brought by the practice of group sex (27 percent stated that they have had group sex). Although 73 percent believe that their behavior puts them at risk for HIV infection, 58 percent never use condoms. Similar to other countries in the region, MSM are largely underground and unorganized (Baran 2002). Although discussions of sexual orientation have become more open in Macedonia, MSM remain highly stigmatized (Wong 2002; IOM and UNICEF 2002). A recent study on MSM conducted by the Center for Human Rights and Conflict Resolution at the Institute for Sociological and Political Legal Research in Skopje found that "a major part of Macedonian citizens consider that homosexuality is an illness of immoral character which is not easily cured... some citizens think that people suffering from this illness should be punished by law" (Macedonia National Multisectoral HIV/AIDS Commission 2003). The RAR found that most young MSM were not well informed about STI/HIV/AIDS. Many stated that they were reluctant to speak openly with their physicians because of stigma (Wong 2002a).

Drug Users. Injecting drug use constitutes the driving force behind the alarming increase in regional HIV/AIDS infection rates. The exact number of injecting drug users in the country is unknown, but, according to Macedonia's Global Fund Coordinating Mechanism, there are an estimated 12,000 to 15,000 IDUs in the country, mostly heroin users. A situation analysis conducted by Macedonia's UN Theme Group on HIV/AIDS estimated that 70 percent of IDUs had hepatitis C (Macedonia Country Coordinating Mechanism 2003), which suggests that IDUs share infected needles.

Apart from unsafe injecting practices, many drug users engage in risk-related sexual behavior, including a cross-over between injecting drug use and commercial sex work. The RAR surveyed two groups of IDUs. In one group, the mean age was 17 years and 55 percent had had sexual intercourse. Of these, 63 percent thought that they were at risk of HIV or other STIs, but only 4 percent percent had been tested for HIV. Approximately 36 percent had between two to five sexual partners in the past year, 43 percent always used condoms during sex, and 8 percent had sex in return for money or drugs (Wong 2002a). In the other group, the mean age was 21 years, and the mean age when drugs were first used was 16 years. Of these, 95 percent had had sexual intercourse, 79 percent thought that they were at risk of HIV or other STIs, and 64 percent percent had been tested for HIV. Almost two-thirds shared drug-injecting equipment, 50 percent had between two and five sexual partners in the past year, 88 percent sometimes or never used condoms during sex, and 25 percent had sex in return for money or drugs.

According to 1999 data published in the 2003 UNODC report, Global Illicit Drug Trends 2003, heroin abuse has increased significantly in Macedonia. Seizures in heroin have increased dramatically, from about 29,000 kilograms in 1996 to 111,000 kilograms in 2001 (this could be due to improved reporting and law enforcement efforts or an increase in trafficking). The Rapid Assessment found that heroin was the most popular drug, followed by marijuana, hashish, methadone, cocaine, ecstasy, LSD and pharmaceuticals. The practice of sharing cooking equipment and loading syringe to syringe is common among IDUs who use drugs in groups, which significantly increases the risk of infection.

IDUs also face a variety of obstacles in accessing treatment options, health insurance, and medical and social services. The UNICEF RAR study found that IDUs are heavily stigmatized and discriminated against by both the general public and medical staff. They do not know where to access health care when needed (Wong 2002a). A strong clinically-oriented approach prevails in interacting with and treating IDUs (IOM and UNICEF 2002).

Prisoners. There are a total of eight prisons in Macedonia housing about 1,500 prisoners, of whom 98 percent are male. There are also special facilities for juveniles. A 2000 report from the Macedonia Clinic for Infectious Diseases, WHO, MOH, and MOJ highlighted that a relatively high percentage of prisoners are drug users involved in high-risk sexual behavior associated with forced and voluntary sex between men. Spreading of Hepatitis C is noticeable among prisoners. Prisoners have poor access to health services and there is a lack of medical staff and available drug treatment. Currently, prisons have no specific HIV prevention programs. However, Macedonia's HIV/AIDS National Strategy 2003–2006 does include programs for prisons: (1) Development and distribution of appropriate education materials; (2) HIV/AIDS inmate peer education activities; and (3) distribution of condoms and lubricants in prisons.

Roma. The Roma community does not have high levels of STIs and HIV, but it is considered a vulnerable group due to a number of inter-related factors. Poverty among the Roma remains one of the most pressing issues for Central and Eastern Europe. In Macedonia, Roma have the lowest socioeconomic status, including low educational and literacy levels. Their general social exclusion restricts their access to information and services (Macedonia National Multisectoral HIV/AIDS Commission 2003; Macedonia CCM 2003). Although some Roma do have access to general HIV/AIDS activities, there are currently no HIV/AIDS programs specifically focused on the Roma community.

HIV/AIDS Awareness and Knowledge

Macedonia's youth, in particular, often have incomplete knowledge about STI and HIV/AIDS and lack the life skills necessary to avoid infection. Even when young people are aware of condoms as a prevention measure for STI/HIV, they fail to use them on a regular basis. Existing health and social services are not youth-friendly and young people reported that they do not obtain information and life skills about sexual health and related issues from their parents or the formal education system.

A survey among 1,200 women in Skopje in 2001 confirmed the existence of a large number of misconceptions about HIV/AIDS and its methods of transmission. A 2002 KAPB survey in Macedonia showed that the share of Albanian and Roma women who said they had open conversations with their children about sexuality and contraception was particularly low. Approximately 37 percent of respondents had not changed their behavior in order to minimize the risk of transmission (MIA 2002).

Considerable stigmatization exists with respect to HIV/AIDS in Macedonia. Additional training and retraining for health providers may be indicated due to the medicalization of HIV and the lack of understanding of the broader health and social aspects. This is particularly relevant to concerns about the lack of confidentiality in the diagnosis and management of HIV/AIDS, with the result that individuals at risk for HIV are reluctant to be tested in Macedonia. Finally, there is often inadequate pre- and post-test counseling and a perception that HIV only has medical implications (Archibald 2002).

Table 28. Knowledge, Attitudes, and Practices—Macedonia

Youth	40% have 2–5 sex partners per year
	40% never or only sometimes use condoms
IDU	95% have sexual intercourse
	51% have between 2–5 sexual partners
MSM	21% have occasional sex
	30% have 5–12 sex partners per year
	58% never use condoms
Juvenile Delinquents	39% IDUs
	74% had sexual intercourse
	24% tested for HIV
	80% "never" or "sometimes" use condoms

Health Care in Macedonia

Before the independence in 1991, the health system in Macedonia resembled that of many other Eastern European countries, offering easy access to comprehensive health care services for the whole population. The system was largely oriented towards curative care, relying on hospitals and specialized polyclinics, while primary and preventive care remained underdeveloped. The system came under increasing pressures, which was exacerbated by the instability in the region with the conflict in Kosovo in 1999 and internal conflict in 2001, as well as the rapid transition to a market economy. Combined with a sharp drop in available public sector resources, the transition has put the financial stability of the health care system under serious strain, and access to care has become increasingly uneven, even after rapid expenditure growth since 1996.

The new Health Insurance Law (April 2000) provides a foundation for some of the reforms needed. An analysis by the European Observatory on Health Care Systems (2002) found that "much of the inherited health care system serves to militate against service efficiency and effectiveness. There is an absence of incentives and a shortage of skills." Priority areas identified for reform include quality of care, service efficiency, cost containment, and equity of provision. The overall strategy is to develop fiscal incentives linked with managerial autonomy and to increase effectiveness of central planning.

Macedonia's health care system is still highly centralized. The Ministry of Health provides central health planning and provides oversight of the national health care system. The national health system has 23,500 employees, of whom 4,500 are physicians. About 60 percent of physicians are employed in primary care. The number of patients per physician varies enormously, however, between 653 and 8,500 (European Observatory on Health Care Systems 2002). There are 18 primary health care centers, 16 medical centers, 7 specialized hospitals, 18 university medical clinics, 16 specialized institutions, and 2 specialized polyclinics. Among governmental health institutions, there are two gynecological clinics. Although many health care institutions are located in relatively new buildings, much of the medical equipment and vehicle stock is outdated or poorly maintained (Wong 2002a). All tertiary care facilities are in the capital, Skopje. The main institution is the Clinical Center, with 18 clinics and institutes and 500 beds. The Ministry of Defense also has military hospitals that provide services free to conscripts and their families.

The Law on Local Self Government envisages decentralization of public health functions. In practice, this might not be possible, and so no real steps have been taken to implement this law. However, the uncertainty created by these provisions has been cited as a reason not to invest further in public health. The Republic Institute of Health Protection is the central institution for public health. Its mandate is to coordinate teaching at the University of Skopje Medical Faculty, supervise and oversee the activities of 10 regional institutes of health protection, and provide technical services to the clinical center and to the country as a whole. The 10 regional institutes have 21 branch offices located in health centers and provide surveillance and hygiene services in the localities (Archibald 2002).

The private health sector in Macedonia is rapidly growing, but it lacks an adequate regulatory framework. Since 2000, there is one private hospital for gynecology and obstetrics (Sistina Medical), but it has no contract with the HIF; and one private hospital for cardio surgery (Philip the Second), which has a contract with the HIF. In addition, there are private medical and dental centers (516 and 377 respectively; Macedonia CCM 2003). The pharmaceutical distribution system was privatized in 1991 and replaced with a system of licensing supervised by the MOH. Public pharmacies contract with the Health Insurance Fund, and dispense drugs from the nationally approved drug list. The Drug Law adopted in 1998 allowed for: (1) streamlined registration of drugs; (2) reference pricing based on generic products; (3) adoption of essential drug lists for public sector reimbursement; and (4) competitive bidding procedures for public sector drug procurement. However, pharmaceutical procurement has been one of the major problems in recent years.

Funding of Health Services

Macedonia's share of overall health expenditure as well as public expenditure as a percentage of GDP is the highest among the countries covered in this study (Table 29). This is also true for the health expenditure per capita, which was US$106 in 2000, more than double the amount in Albania. Yet, although Macedonia's health spending is more or less in line with the regional average, a worsening financial situation has led to problems with equity and access to health services, especially for the poor and vulnerable groups.

Funding for HIV/AIDS

The total necessary funding for the implementation of the national HIV/AIDS Strategy for 2003–2006 is estimated at US$12 million. According to the National Strategy, the public budget for HIV/AIDS is projected to increase from US$95,474 in 2003 to $236,082 in 2006. In terms of percentage of the total health budget, the share of funds for the prevention of HIV/AIDS would thus double from 0.63 percent of the total Government health budget in 2004 to 1.12 percent in 2006. The National Multisectoral HIV/AIDS Commission (2003) notes, however, that "this budget increase is ambitious given the current economic

Table 29. Health Expenditure and GDP Trends in Macedonia 1990–2001

	1990	1995	1996	1997	1998	1999	2000	2001
Health expenditure per capita (current US$)	—	119	129	114	135	107	106	—
Health expenditure, private (% of GDP)	0	0.49	0.75	0.98	0.98	0.94	0.93	—
Health expenditure, public (% of GDP)	9.19	4.71	5.05	5.12	6.62	4.96	5.07	—
Health expenditure, total (% of GDP)	9.19	5.2	5.8	6.1	7.6	5.9	6	—
GDP per capita, PPP (current international $)	5,829	5,454	5,543	5,582	5,686	6,028	6,508	6,232
GDP growth (annual %)	—	−1.11	1.18	1.4	3.4	4.32	4.55	−4.53

Source: World Bank HNP Stats Database.

uncertainties." The National Health Insurance Fund budgeted an additional $84,418 for HIV/AIDS, and the Global Fund (GFATM) has granted $4.4 million for a period of two years (2004–2006). According to the grant proposal, expected additional funds from other sources amount to around $1.1 million over a five-year period.

The overall level of public funding was below needs before the GFATM grant award. The HIV/AIDS program is funded from the budget through a reimbursement system that takes into account output. The Health Insurance Fund pays for drugs, and limited interventions related to testing and counseling. In principle, patients with HIV/AIDS are covered by the HIF, either through employment or through transfers for the unemployed from the Employment Bureau to the HIF. HIV patients are exempted from the 20 percent co-payment, and receive free treatment from the Institute of Infectious Diseases.

Problems have been reported with regard to the availability of public budgeted funds, particularly for prevention measures, and the actual level of spending was below budget targets. However, serious access problems have been reported. The reimbursement rates are well below market costs, and do not provide an incentive for the Institute of Infectious Diseases and the IPHs to expand their public health services, particularly in the areas of testing and counseling. Public funding provided for treatment of HIV/AIDS in the HIF budget only covered expenditure for treatment of five patients. On the other hand, costs for drug treatment and HIF drug reimbursement are exceeding international levels: the Skopje Center—its center for prevention and treatment of drug use—provides methadone treatment for approximately 150–200 drug users, which would cost $400–500 per year per patient, as compared to US$70 at international market prices.

Resource Gap

Overall funding needs for HIV/AIDS in Macedonia have been estimated between $3.9 and $5.1 million for the period from 2003 to 2006.[10] By comparing anticipated funding levels with the total resource estimate for Macedonia, it could be assumed that funding needs would almost be covered in 2004 through the GFATM, and a gap in later years would be less severe than in neighboring countries. However, the epidemiological situation suggests that the number of HIV/AIDS infected people is very likely to be substantially higher than assumed in the projections used for calculation of the funding requirements in the GFATM proposal. This means that in addition to urgently needed policy changes to reduce treatment cost (particularly for HAART), it would be necessary to substantially increase domestic funding and resource mobilization at much higher levels than envisaged at present.

Government and Civil Society Action on HIV/AIDS

Strategic, Policy, and Regulatory Framework

Macedonia established its first AIDS program in 1985, two years prior to the first reported HIV infection. In 1987, the National HIV/AIDS Program began to be implemented

---

10. A recent study of the UNAIDS and The World Bank (2003) has estimated the total funding requirement to effectively combat HIV/AIDS in the countries in the region until 2007. These estimates cover resource needs for comprehensive care (including HAART) and prevention programs.

Table 30. Estimated Resource Needs and Funding Gaps for HIV/AIDS Treatment—Macedonia

Macedonia ('000 US$)	2001	2002	2003	2004	2005	2006
Available and planned HIV/AIDS Funding (2)						
Government allocation		170	226	269	328	405
Central budget		85	111	149	202	272
Health Insurance Fund		85	115	120	126	133
Domestic Other		364	364	364	364	364
Donor allocation		810	810	810	810	810
Requested from GFATM				2,442	1,907	1,961
Estimated total HIV/AIDS resource needs (1)	4,193	4,031	3,891	4,063	4,463	5,132
Funding gap		2,686	2,491	1,789	1,054	1,592

Source: 1. WB/UNAIDS estimates, 2. GFATM proposal.

through the National AIDS Committee under the MOH, with a national AIDS coordinator as the focal point. A UN Theme Group on HIV/AIDS (UNTG) has been active in Macedonia since 1999. The UN Theme Group is currently chaired by UNDP and composed of UNICEF, WHO, IOM, UNHCR, and the World Bank. In 2003, UNICEF chaired the Technical Working Group (TWG), and works together with the National HIV/AIDS Coordinator and non-governmental organizations. In June 2001, the country signed the Declaration of Commitment on HIV/AIDS adopted in New York at the UN General Assembly Special Session on HIV/AIDS (UNGASS).

In April 2003, the National Multisectoral HIV/AIDS Commission (NMC) succeeded the National HIV/AIDS Committee. This Commission expands on the previous medical focus of the National HIV/AIDS Committee to include members from other ministries and sectors. The NMC comprises 28 members, including representatives from the ministries of Health, Interior, Justice, Finance, Education, Labor, and Local Self Government; NGOs; religious organizations; academic institutions; medical services; and the UN Theme Group on HIV/AIDS. The Ministry of Health acts as the Secretariat to the NMC through administrative staff nominated by the State Secretary of Health.

In July 2003, the National Multisectoral HIV/AIDS Commission approved the Macedonia HIV/AIDS National Strategy 2003–2006. The Strategy was designed as a framework to guide development, implementation, monitoring, and evaluation of HIV/AIDS-focused programming in the national context. Accession to the European Union presents an additional strong incentive for FYR Macedonia to implement an appropriate strategy for HIV/AIDS. Some of the priorities identified in the National Strategy are:

- Preventing the spread of HIV/AIDS among vulnerable groups (youth, IDUs, sex workers, MSM, mobile groups, Roma, and prisoners)
- Improving access to, and the quality of, counselling and testing services
- Improving national epidemiological and behavioural surveillance systems

▧ Improving the provision of care and support for PLWHA
▧ Preventing HIV transmission in health care settings
▧ Strengthening capacity and coordination within the national response to HIV/AIDS

The GFATM approved a grant of $4.3 million over two years for the National Strategy. The grant proposal has 10 objectives. The first six focus on preventing HIV among vulnerable groups, including youth, IDUs, sex workers, MSM, Roma, and prisoners. Expected results include increasing the number of members of vulnerable groups that are reached with targeted HIV/AIDS interventions in three years, for example, increasing IDUs reached from 2,680 to 6,500; sex workers from 103 to 250; MSM from 250 to 750; and reaching 21,300 Roma and 1,500 prisoners for whom there are currently no HIV/AIDS interventions.

The GFATM grant application, boosted cooperation among key stakeholders in the country. Coordination between different sectors, Ministries and services involved on HIVAIDS, STIs and TB control has improved since the establishment of the Country Coordination Mechanism. It enabled the establishment of a missing link between Government organizations and NGOs, and supports the development of harm reduction approaches to decrease vulnerability of drug users to HIV/AIDS. However, the Republican Institute for Health Protection and the Clinic for Infectious Diseases, two key health institutions, have only recently been integrated into the overall planning process and implementation of the National AIDS Strategy.

Table 31. Government Intervention and Institutional Arrangements—Macedonia

Intersectoral coordination	▧ National Multisectoral HIV/AIDS Commission (NMC) has been established
	▧ National GFATM Coordination Mechanism has been established
	▧ Inter-Ministerial National Commission to Combat Human Trafficking established
	▧ UN Theme Group on HIV/AIDS (UNTG) is functional
National HIV/AIDS Strategy and Legislation	▧ National HIV/AIDS Strategy 2003–2006 has been developed
	▧ 2000 PRSP does not mention HIV/AIDS
	▧ Agreement on Cooperation to Prevent and Combat Transborder Crime has been ratified
	▧ Protocol to Prevent, Suppress and Punish Trafficking of People has been signed
	▧ Anti-Trafficking National Plan of Action (NPA) is developed
	▧ National HIV/AIDS Strategy for 2003–2006 has an estimated cost of $12 million
Government institution responsible for HIV/AIDS	▧ GFATM grant of $4.3 million has been awarded
	▧ National AIDS Committee under MOH
	▧ Republican Institute of Health Protection in Skopje is the central institution for public health. Has 10 regional Institutes and 21 branch offices

Macedonia has already initiated a review of the legal framework focused on HIV/AIDS issues, including people living with AIDS. Each year, the Macedonian government formulates a program for HIV/AIDS control and control of communicable diseases, including STIs, according to the proposal put forward by the Macedonian MOH. The priorities are education, prevention and treatment. However, treatment with antiretroviral drugs is not available. Macedonia's Global Fund Country Coordination Mechanism, which has been established to apply for GFATM grant funding, reports that to date HIV/AIDS activities have been small-scale, uncoordinated, and sporadic. Interventions targeting vulnerable subpopulations (including youth, IDUs, sex workers, MSM, prisoners, and Roma) have been negligible. Other key gaps include:

- High levels of HIV/AIDS-related stigma and discrimination.
- The Parliament is considering decriminalization of CSW, but legislation regarding NGOs is necessary.
- PLWHA should be included in the NMC; and the relative roles of the CCM and NMC have to be clarified.
- Limited availability of key serological and behavioral surveillance data.
- Need for expanded harm reduction and drug treatment programs for IDUs.
- Limited access to VCT, with existing services of variable quality.
- Limited access to medical care and support for PLWHA.
- Relatively limited capacity to address HIV/AIDS.
- Fragmentation of services and approaches.

In addition, in 1999, the Macedonian Government ratified the Agreement on Cooperation to Prevent and Combat Transborder Crime with SECI. MOI is working with SECI on developing intelligence sharing and a trans-national database. In December 2000, Macedonia became a signatory to the UN Protocol to Prevent, Suppress and Punish Trafficking of People. In 2001, an Inter-Ministerial National Commission to Combat Human Trafficking was established chaired by the Ministry of the Interior State Secretary. This Commission drafted and adopted an Anti-Trafficking National Plan of Action (NPA).

HIV/AIDS and STIs Surveillance

CIDA has recently funded a Rapid Assessment of the Macedonia HIV/AIDS and STI surveillance system, which provides the most exhaustive, up-to date information. The information presented in this section is drawn from this Rapid Assessment (Archibald 2002). According to the assessment, the surveillance system of FYR Macedonia has a solid foundation and potential to provide useful information for public health action. However, low reporting of STIs, low number of registered IDUs, and other deficiencies in the system suggest serious weaknesses of the surveillance system. There is no sentinel surveillance for risk groups, and the existing HIV case reporting system has serious limitations. Given the lack of national HIV seroprevalence and formal behavioral surveillance studies, the ability to discern dynamics and trends in HIV/AIDS in Macedonia is highly constrained. Also, the atmosphere of stigma and discrimination surrounding HIV/AIDS makes it difficult for individuals to admit to certain risk behaviors, which gives a bias to the information collected, especially concerning risk groups. Confidentiality concerns spur some Macedonians to opt for HIV testing abroad, thereby weakening the reporting system for HIV. The procedures

Table 32. Government Intervention and Institutional Arrangements—Macedonia

Testing	
	▓ GFATM grant aims at increasing the annual number of those being tested voluntarily for HIV from the current 250 to 1000 within 3 years
	▓ Testing is free with a doctor's referral, otherwise costs around 20 Euros
	▓ ELISA testing for HIV is available at 4 public facilities
	▓ Confirmation tests are provided at the Clinic of Infectious Diseases (CID)
	▓ Few private clinics in Skopje have kits for HIV testing
	▓ Rapid tests are not available
	▓ No pre and post-test counseling is offered at these facilities
Surveillance	▓ Serious weaknesses in the surveillance system
	▓ Atmosphere of stigma and discrimination around HIV/AIDS prevents individuals from admitting risk behavior
HIV/AIDS Notification	▓ Roles and responsibilities of different institutions in notification are not well defined
Blood Safety	▓ The Institute of Transfusion ensures national coordination of blood donation
	▓ All donated blood products undergo mandatory testing for HIV
	▓ 48,000–50,000 blood units tested each year
	▓ Donated blood is tested 3 times by using the same testing methods
Prevention	▓ Limited prevention activities until obtaining GFATM grant
Treatment	▓ The Health Insurance Fund pays for drugs. HIV patients are exempted from 20% co-payment
	▓ Public funds could cover only 5 patients
	▓ ARV drugs are not available

to guide HIV/AIDS and STI surveillance, as well as roles and responsibilities of different institutions in reporting are not well defined.

As in other countries, surveillance needs to be established. However, this has not been included under the GFATM grant, so additional funding has to be identified for this activity. Monitoring and evaluation are being developed under the GFATM grant, but a M&E plan and indicators that allow for comparisons with other countries have to be adopted.

In addition to the aforementioned goals of Macedonia's National HIV/AIDS Strategy, the Strategy also seeks to develop a national policy on HIV testing, specifically an accessible, voluntary, confidential HIV testing system that includes pre- and post-test counseling. The Strategy's target interventions include:

▓ Ensure availability of voluntary HIV testing, including anonymous testing, to include pre- and post-test counseling.

▓ Develop guidelines for public and private institutions (including NGOs) to standardize testing and counseling procedures.

- ▓ Provide the necessary resources (human and financial) to secure an appropriate pre- and post-test counseling system.
- ▓ Inform the public about testing procedures, sites and rights.

One of the objectives of Macedonia's GFATM grant is to increase the annual number of those being tested voluntarily for HIV from the current 250 to 1,000 within three years. Available HIV data are based on test results in limited settings, including primarily blood/organ donor sites. In fact, almost all reported HIV cases were only tested for HIV after they had had health problems. Most developed full-blown AIDS six to 12 months after testing, indicating that their status was discovered late in the course of the disease (Macedonia National Multisectoral HIV/AIDS Commission 2003).

ELISA testing for HIV is available at four public facilities: Clinic for Infectious Diseases (CID); Institute of Clinical Biochemistry; Republic Institute for Health Protection; and Institute for Transfusion. However, sustaining supplies is a problem due to lack of resources. Confirmation tests are carried out at the Clinic for Infectious Diseases (CID), where the Western Blot test is used. In the capital Skopje, there are a few private laboratories, which have kits for HIV, but other parts of Macedonia do not have access to testing. Rapid tests are also available over the counter. There are no quality assurance programs in place for either the laboratories performing the HIV screening tests or the central laboratory performing the confirmatory test (Archibald 2002; IOM and UNICEF 2002).

The European AIDS case definition is used, and data are reported to the European Center for the Epidemiological Monitoring of AIDS (EuroHIV) in France. However, the Assessment of HIV/AIDS/STI surveillance in Macedonia noted that it is not clear whether physicians understand this definition and use it appropriately, partly because Macedonia has limited diagnostic equipment for AIDS. As of late 2002, the role of the National AIDS Coordinator (NAC), based at the Institute of Epidemiology and Biostatistics, was not clearly defined. This position has a role in addressing HIV prevention, reporting to the National Multisectoral HIV/AIDS Commission, and in dealing with the media, but the role regarding data analysis, interpretation, and dissemination is not clear (Archibald 2002).

HIV testing is free with a doctor's referral; otherwise, the cost is approximately 20 Euros. Generally, the four official testing facilities do not offer HIV counseling; the limited pre- and post-test counseling available is provided by NGOs. Uptake of VCT is hindered by stigma and concerns regarding confidentiality. The National Multisectoral HIV/AIDS Commission (2003) reports that some Macedonians opt for HIV testing abroad because of these concerns.

STIs are not regularly or reliably reported and are seriously under-reported. By law, it is obligatory to report cases of syphilis and gonorrhea to the Republic Institute for Health Protection. According to the medical staff in charge of the diagnosis of chlamydia, genital herpes, and other STIs, the number of cases is increasing very rapidly, especially among the younger population. There is recognition among public health professionals that the low number of reported STI cases does not represent the reality. Rather, the low numbers are a consequence of poor surveillance, break down in the reporting system, increase of self-medication, and poor access to basic services. The reporting system for both private and governmental institutions is weak and passive. There are no incentives for providers to report infectious diseases nor there is a strict mechanism of control of reporting from the central level.

It is believed that many doctors do not report syphilis according to established proce-dures, and that doctors in private clinics are much less likely to report cases. Gonorrhea is even less likely to be reported since it is generally not taken as seriously as syphilis by the medical profession. An additional aspect leading to the under-reporting of STIs is that patients often ask not to be reported since their name and address appear on the reporting form. There is also a lot of self-diagnosis and self-treatment for STIs, since antibiotics can easily be obtained without a doctor's prescription. There is no requirement to report STIs such as herpes or chlamydia, and little data exist on these diseases.

Laboratory diagnoses of STIs are carried out in the Department for Epidemiology within the National Public Health Institute. Limited STI testing is also available in the ten regional Institutes for Public Health. Although an official accreditation body does not exist, all laboratories are recognized and nominated by the Ministry of Health on the basis of criteria for space, equipment, and staff availability. The Department for Epidemiology and Microbiology sends tabular STI data to WHO in Copenhagen and also to the National Coordinator for Infectious Diseases in the Institute of Epidemiology and Biostatistics.

The National Institute of Transfusiology ensures national coordination of blood dona-tion. Since 1997, all donated blood products have undergone mandatory testing for HIV. Blood is also tested for Hepatitis B and C and syphilis. A few years ago, the Blood transfu-sion service used ELISA test kits for syphilis, but the Institute can no longer afford these kits. Approximately 48,000–50,000 blood units are tested each year. Since 1974, blood donation has been voluntary. Donors do not receive material compensation, however, those who donate over 10 times receive minor benefits (Macedonia National Multisectoral HIV/AIDS Commission 2003).

HIV/AIDS and STIs Prevention and Control in the Public System

Universal precautions are not well understood in Macedonia's health system. Most health institutions have no specific instructions on HIV precautions for their staff. The government has not provided any guidelines. Moreover, the availability of equipment required to comply with UP is not guaranteed. However, the GFATM grant provides sufficient funds for the Government to initiate prevention activities in 2004. In addi-tion to the priorities already mentioned, the National HIV/AIDS Strategy also sets out the following:

- Ensure that all pregnant women receive adequate counseling about the risks of HIV/AIDS, and that they have access to VCT.
- Ensure standard protocol and resources for routine HAART are made available to all pregnant women found to be HIV-positive.
- Ensure health staff has the skills and knowledge to comply with counseling and testing procedures and ensure confidentiality.

However, PMTCT is not mentioned in the March 2003 GFATM proposal (Macedonia CCM 2003). Sex education in schools has not yet been systematically developed. Health professionals throughout the country are poorly informed about HIV/AIDS diagnosis and treatment, and sometimes have little or no access to protective equipment.

HIV/AIDS and STIs Treatment

Treatment for opportunistic infections is only available through the AIDS Clinic at the Infectious Diseases Hospital in Skopje. PLWHA are followed clinically every three to six months at CID. No PCR or viral load testing is done in Macedonia. Local CD4 testing only provides relative and not absolute cell counts (Archibald 2002). The Department for HIV/AIDS at the CID offers limited space for AIDS patients, but cannot offer full-time antiretroviral therapy. The National AIDS Commission and Ministry of Health decided in 2003 that registration of ARV drugs would be free of charge as an incentive for pharmaceutical companies to register these drugs. Clinical care is free although the patient must pay for transportation to CID. Clinical guidelines and protocols of treatment, care and support for PLWHA have been prepared.

The approach to STI prevention and control in Macedonia is clinically-based, operating within 12 specialist clinics throughout the country. Nine of these are out-patient centers for STI diagnoses and treatment that function as a part of larger health centers: five are located within major primary health centers in Skopje and four within secondary health centers in Bitola, Ohrid, Prilep, and Stip. Training in dermatovenerology and in infectious diseases is available in the country and is required for practicing STI and HIV/AIDS treatment respectively. Each is a three-year program involving theoretical and practical components; these training programs are currently reported to be undergoing harmonization with EU programs. The university hospital in Skopje is also a center for education and research in the area of STIs.

The Center for prevention and treatment of addition, which is part of the Psychiatric Hospital in Skopje, provides methadone treatment for 320 drug users.

Decentralized community care and social support are underdeveloped or provided on an ad hoc basis. One of the objectives of Macedonia's GFATM grant is to provide health care and psychosocial support for PLWHA. It is anticipated that at least 20 PLWHA will be receiving ARVs within three years. In its budget, the GFATM proposal cites the annual cost of ARVs at US$1,181. In this area, Macedonia's National HIV/AIDS Strategy includes:

- Support the development of standard guidelines for palliative care.
- Support clinical management training for health workers.
- Support the development of civil society capacity to provide alternative care and support services for PLWHA.
- Develop the capacity of general practitioners to provide basic medical and counseling services to PLWHA.
- Develop and implement a standard national protocol for treatment and care of PLWHA.
- Include a minimum of seven HAART drugs on the drug list reimbursed by the Health Insurance Fund.
- Ensure that adequate resources are allocated, so that all people with HIV/AIDS have equal access to the defined standard treatment and to treatment for OIs.
- Provide training to health professionals on the clinical management of AIDS, with particular focus on HAART.

Table 33. NGO Sector in Macedonia

▨ Center for Human Rights and Conflict Resolution: MSM study

▨ HELP Gostivar: Established new harm reduction programs including development of special services for sex workers who are IDUs

▨ HERA: Established pilot educational center for HIV/AIDS/STI and reproductive health. Has an AIDS help and information telephone line as well as a peer education program for MSM. Has created a network within Macedonia and abroad for the provision of assistance involving treatment, information on new developments, and financial support for PLWHA (IOM and UNICEF 2002; Archibald 2002).

▨ HOPS is the only organization providing harm reduction services to IDUs and sex workers, including needle exchange, outreach counseling and an SOS hotline. HOPS also plays an advocacy role and is involved in a program to decentralize substitution therapy. HOPS workers access IDUs via outreach work and also through needle exchange sites. With support from OSI, HOPS also works with street-based sex workers in Skopje. It distributes condoms and aids in developing condom negotiation skills.

▨ The Macedonian Interethnic Association (MIA) has created a network related to AIDS awareness, human rights, and support for PLWHA. It runs an AIDS information telephone line, and with EU funding, has collaborated with a Bulgarian NGO to reach young Roma girls who were at risk of becoming sex workers. MIA has also conducted several KAP studies (IOM and UNICEF 2002).

▨ The Macedonian Medical Students Association (MMSA) is forming networks for peer education and is expanding its activities in primary and high schools. MMSA is developing a program to support HIV training for medical students.

▨ TRUST (Association for the Improvement of Treatment, Rehabilitation and Resocialization of Drug Users) is promoting regular HIV testing among drug users. TRUST is also actively involved in lobbying for substitution therapy.

▨ IOM is actively involved in the repatriation of trafficked women. It also provides HIV testing for emigration candidates if required by country of destination.

▨ The Open Society Institute supports needle exchange and harm reduction programs with IDUs.

▨ Through RiskNet, funded by USAID, PSI supports NGOs engaging in harm reduction activities, including referrals to treatment centers; VCT; and distribution of condoms, clean needles (not funded by USAID), and educational materials. In addition, RiskNet has conducted both peer ethnographic research among MSM and NGO workshops to develop effective outreach activities that reduce stigma and discrimination (Population Services International 2003).

▨ Other NGOs are also providing some services to sex workers on a small scale (103 sex workers were reached with targeted HIV/AIDS interventions during 2002; Macedonia CCM 2003).

Table 34. World Bank Support—Macedonia

Projects that address HIV directly	Projects that could include HIV/AIDS action	Analytical work that addresses HIV or risk factors
	Trade and Transport Facilitation in Southeast Europe	
	Transport Sector	
	Children and Youth Development	
	Education Modernization	
	Social Protection	
	Health and other social services	
	Health Sector Management Project	

HIV/AIDS Prevention and Control by NGOs

FYR Macedonia has experienced the emergence of a small, but effective NGO community that works closely with vulnerable groups. These include HOPS, HERA, MIA, DOVERBA, MMSA, and Passage. There are also several international NGOs. NGOs carry out a wide range of outreach activities. Consequently, many people from vulnerable sub-populations find services offered by NGOs to be readily accessible to them. This is particularly important in the current environment, where many people from vulnerable groups find themselves subject to considerable stigma and discrimination. However, the NGO sector is relatively new in FYR Macedonia. There is need for these NGOs to develop further institutional capacity, to work more cooperatively with each other, to facilitate the development of services outside the capital, and to establish sustainable funding (Macedonia CCM 2003). Macedonian NGOs report dwindling financial support, mainly due to a reduction in donor activities, after high levels of funding following the 2001 Peace Accord. This funding gap may need to be covered by either Government sources or increased fund raising by the NGOs.

The Government needs to recognize the role and comparative advantage of NGOs, which would require difficult institutional changes within key Government health institutions. Although a registration and legal framework for NGOs was established in 1999, financial regulations for NGOs are not clear. This applies particularly to the treatment of limited income-generating activities on the part of some NGOs. NGOs (as well as the public sector) are in need of training to improve their project implementation and financial management skills.

International Partner Organizations

Generally, donor funding for HIV has dropped over the last years in the region. Many international donors are reducing their activities, or even closing their local offices. With World Bank funding of US$750,000 during 1996–2000, Macedonia purchased TB X-ray and laboratory equipment. The new Bank-financed health project focus on strenghtening the management of the Health Insurance Fund, and could contribute to improving allocation of funds for HIV/AIDS.

Table 35. International Support—Macedonia

UNTG	■ The UN Theme Group on HIV/AIDS has been active in Macedonia since November1999
	■ UNTG has assisted the preparation of the National HIV/AIDS Strategy
	■ In 2002–2003, $98,000 from the Program Accelerating Funds (PAF) financed strategic planning process in the country and supports the GFATM application
UNAIDS	■ UNAIDS assisted the development of the national strategic process, GFATM application and M&E system
GFATM	■ Provided $4.4 million for TB and HIV/AIDS
UNICEF	■ Awareness raising and social mobilization on risks and prevention
	■ Supports peer and life skills education
	■ Undertook rapid assessment of youth (RAR)
	■ Collaborates with Ministry of Interior on anti-trafficking activities
	■ Supports local SOS help-line to inform and prevent girls and women from being trafficked
	■ Strengthens capacity of government and NGOs to adopt and implement special protection measures for child victims of trafficking
	■ Increases capacity of pedagogues and psychologists and Centers for Social Work to provide psychosocial support and abuse awareness leading to better referral mechanisms between schools, centers for social work and local NGOs
UNDP	■ UNDP has assisted the formulation of the National HIV/AIDS Strategy.
	■ Strengthening institutional capacities for planning and implementation of multi-sectoral strategies to limit the spread of HIV/AIDS and mitigate its social and economic impact
WHO	■ Collaborates with MOH to support blood transfusion services
	■ Has provided training for health professionals in HIV/AIDS prevention
	■ Published and disseminated 20,000 copies of "HIV/AIDS Prevention Guidelines for Health Workers" across the country
	■ Supported study of prisons, drug use, and sexual behavior in 2001
	■ Provides assistance on TB control
OSCE	■ Hosts anti-trafficking training workshops and seminars targeting government officials, legal community and law enforcement agents
	■ Funds Trafficked Victim SOS Helpline
	■ Provides anti-trafficking technical expertise and support to the inter-ministerial National Commission to Combat Trafficking, Ministries of Interior and Justice, Police Academy and others
	■ Implements specialized training on gender and human trafficking targeting police officers and police cadets
	■ Funds preventive gender projects for raising awareness of domestic violence in Roma communities countrywide
	■ Supports Office of Human Rights Ombudsman
SIDA US$455,000	■ Preventive activities
	■ Finances Project Hope prevention, and care and support activities

(*continued*)

Table 35. International Support—Macedonia (*Continued*)

NORAD US$25,000	▨ Supports Ministry of Interior's Center for Trafficked Persons ▨ Supports gender activities of Ministry of Labor and Social Policy
CIDA	▨ Supports IOM anti-trafficking activities
USAID US$200,000	▨ Rapid Assessment of HIV/AIDS and STI Surveillance System ▨ Strengthening NGO capacity in voluntary counseling and testing ▨ Special Initiatives and Cross-Cutting Programs (FY03 US$8.9 million, 20%) ▨ Addresses issues such as ethnic cooperation; gender-based problems and disparities; problems that affect youth; corruption; and needs that are identified for specialized training outside Macedonia ▨ Social marketing program with Population Services International (PSI) ▨ Co-financed the preparation of the GFATM proposal ▨ Supports Ministry of Interior's Center for Trafficked Persons and IOM anti-trafficking activities ▨ Funds Institute for Sustainable Communities targeting local NGOs working on anti-trafficking and public health

CHAPTER 9

Profile: Serbia

Table 36. Epidemiology—Serbia

Population **Census 2002**	7.5 million
Registered HIV cases	1,912
Registered AIDS cases IPH 2004	1,244
HIV/AIDS Prevalence UNAIDS 2003	<0.1
New HIV Cases IPH 2004	101
Modes of Transmission IPH 2004	Heterosexual 24% Homosexual 30% IDU 14% Unknown 26% Blood 3%
Registered STIs cases Federal IHP 2004	MTC 3% Syphilis: 1,232 (1992–2003)
TB notification rate Federal IHP 2003	Gonorrhea: 5,213 (1992–2003) 37/100,000

(*continued*)

Table 36. Epidemiology—Serbia (*Continued*)

Vulnerable Groups	Youth
UNICEF RAR 2002	▓ 20% of population under 15
	IDU
	▓ Estimated number 100,000
	▓ HIV prevalence rate 1.7%
	▓ 62% do not consider drug use to be risk factor
	▓ 57% share needles
	▓ 95% have sex
	▓ 30% never use condoms
	▓ 37% positive for Hepatitis C
	▓ 34% tested for HIV
	CSW
	▓ Estimated number 3,000 in Belgrade
	▓ Mean age 21
	▓ 57% used drugs
	▓ Are paid if not using condoms
	▓ 57% tested for HIV
	MSM
	▓ HIV prevalence rate 2.3%
	▓ 77% use drugs
	▓ 61% always use condoms
	▓ 41% tested for HIV
	▓ Highly stigmatized and discriminated

Epidemiological Overview

HIV/AIDS

From 1984 through the end of 2004, there were 1,912 HIV infections reported in Serbia. At the beginning of the epidemic, the ratio between men and women was 5:1 among newly diagnosed cases, whereas in 2003 it was 3:1. In the first decade of the HIV epidemic, 70 percent of HIV cases were traced to IDU. Since 1994, most known HIV cases were associated with sexual transmission, and only 14 percent of all new infections in 2003 were among IDUs. The "unknown route of transmission" (18 percent in 2003, 9 percent overall) shows an increasing trend among mostly men, similar to that of homo/bisexual transmission, suggesting that a significant proportion of MSM transmission is unreported probably because of the strong stigmatization of this group. The most affected group was in the age range of 30–39 (38 percent), and primarily men (71 percent).

Geographically, the majority of reported HIV cases (84 percent) were from Belgrade. From 1987 through June 2002, there have been a total of 1,419 HIV infections registered there. Out of a total of 1,720 cases, and 103 new infections in 2002, the Belgrade

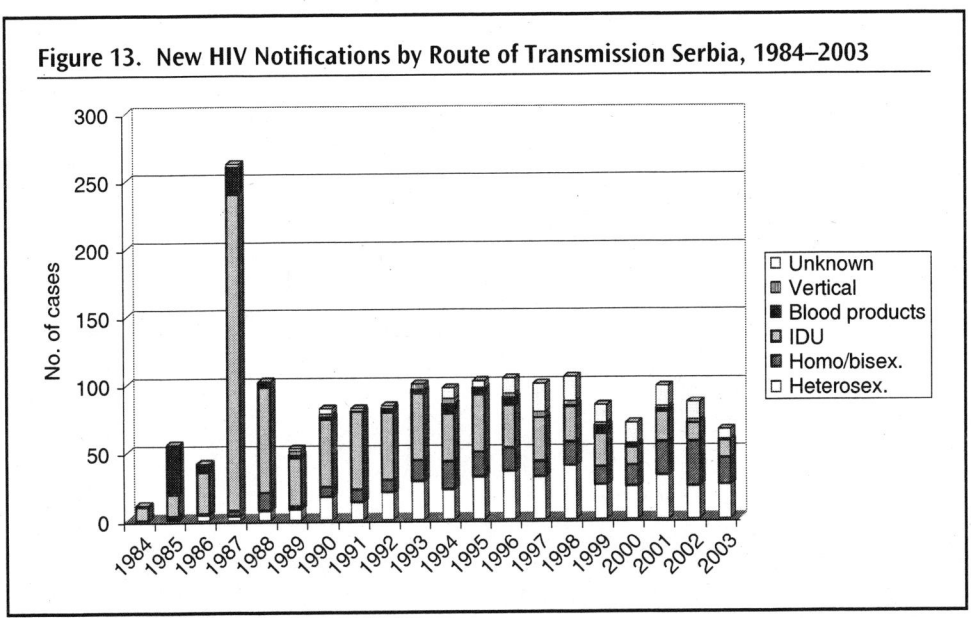

Figure 13. New HIV Notifications by Route of Transmission Serbia, 1984–2003

Source: IPH Serbia 2003.

IPH reported 43 new HIV infections, most aged between 20 and 39 years and associated with sexual transmission (40 percent heterosexual; 26 percent homosexual). Whereas 19 percent of registered HIV infections were among IDUs in 2002, 63 percent were among IDUs 10 years earlier (Rhodes and others 2003). In 2004, 60 of the 101 reported new cases were in Belgrade.

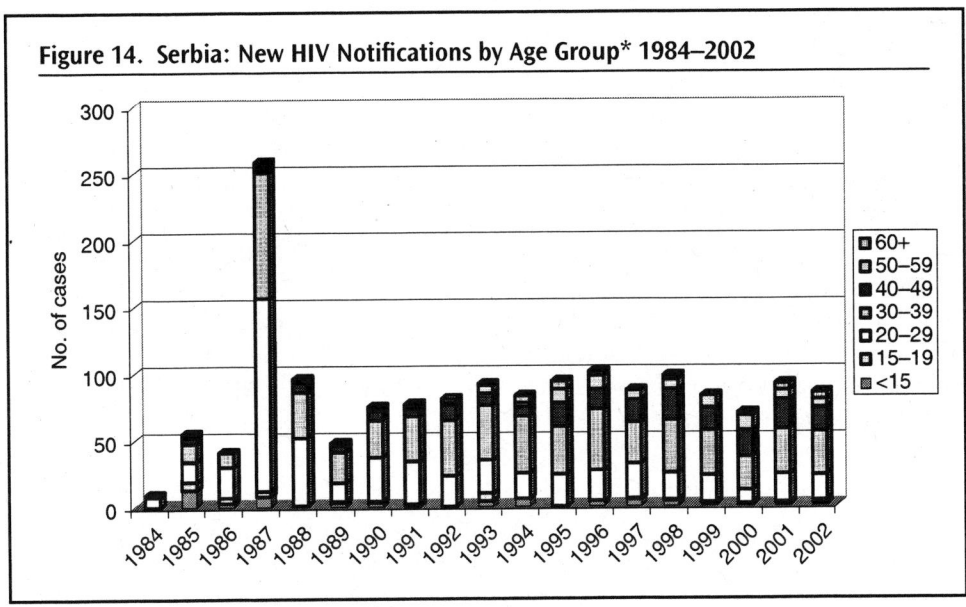

Figure 14. Serbia: New HIV Notifications by Age Group* 1984–2002

*75 cases had unknown age.
Source: IPH Serbia 2003.

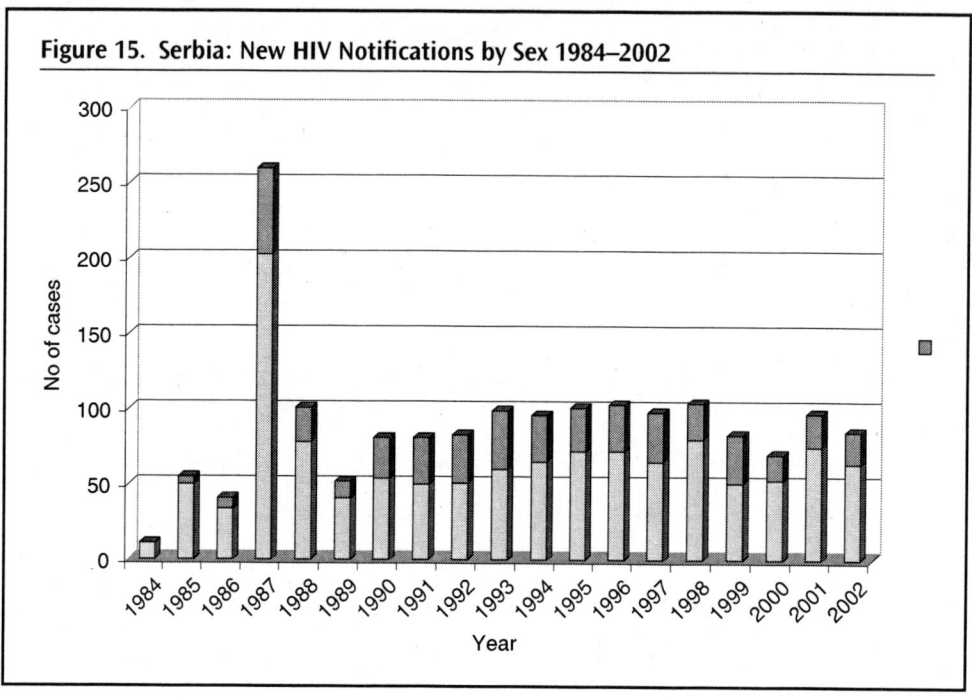

Figure 15. Serbia: New HIV Notifications by Sex 1984–2002

Source: IPH Serbia 2003.

The first HIV infection in Yugoslavia was identified in 1984. The first two cases of AIDS in Yugoslavia were reported in 1985. All official data on HIV/AIDS are reported to the WHO and EURO/HIV. There is, however, a deficiency of routine data on HIV infection among vulnerable populations. The most comprehensive research to date among vulnerable populations is the Rapid Assessment and Response (RAR) studies sponsored by UNICEF. The RAR studies show reported HIV prevalence among IDU and MSM to be 1.7 percent and 2.3 percent respectively. No HIV data are provided for commercial sex workers (CSWs), but reported STI infections are comparatively higher among CSWs. Since these reports reflect only a few cases among the risk groups surveyed, the true HIV prevalence is undoubtedly higher.

DFID has noted in the report *HIV Prevention Among Vulnerable Populations Initiative in Serbia and Montenegro* that the apparent decline in HIV infection among IDUs may be due to limited surveillance of both HIV incidence and IDUs (Rhodes and others 2003). Moreover, the Initiative's July 2003 report suggested that HIV testing programs previously targeted drug injectors in Serbia. Many of the more established older injectors known to authorities had histories of HIV testing, whereas younger IDUs were less likely to be tested. Additionally, the proportion of IDUs tested for HIV may have declined over time. Since 1993, for example, less than 10 percent of newly admitted drug users to the Institute of Dependence Diseases have been tested for HIV, indicating that it is almost impossible to establish trends for HIV among IDUs. The European Center for the Epidemiological Monitoring of AIDS (EuroHIV) has reported HIV/AIDS data for Serbia and Montenegro, though not disaggregated by republic.

In Serbia, there were 1,244 AIDS cases reported through the end of 2004; of them, 871 have died. Over 80 percent of reported AIDS cases are from Belgrade. Overall, 73 percent

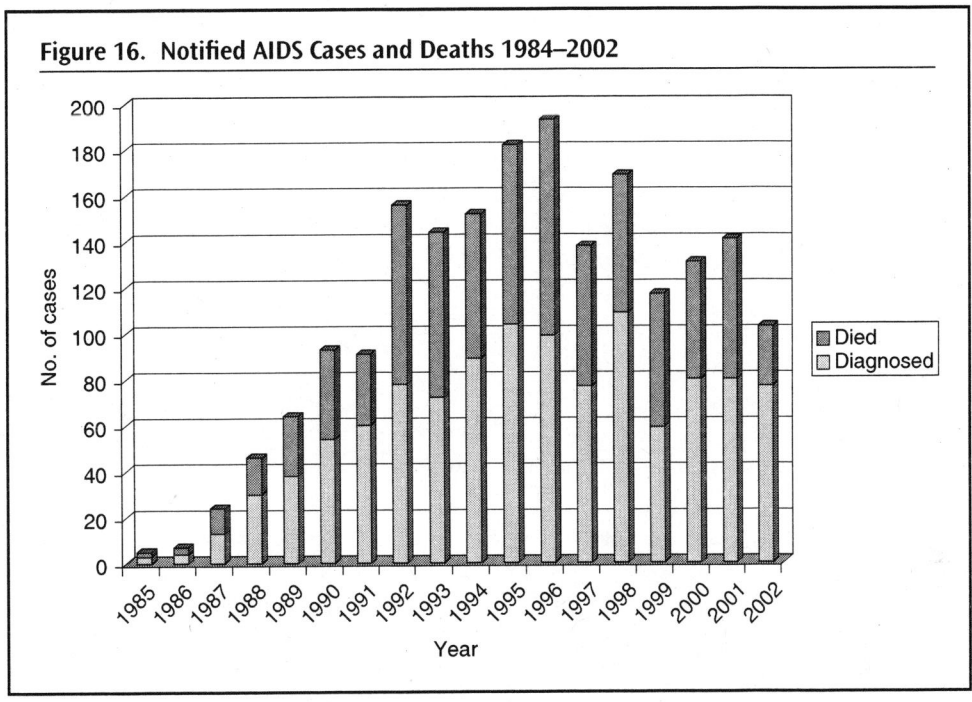

Figure 16. Notified AIDS Cases and Deaths 1984–2002

Source: IPH Serbia 2003.

of AIDS cases are male, although the number of cases among women was higher between 1997 and 2001. Over 80 percent of AIDS cases are among people aged 20 to 49 years, and 48 percent are among people aged 30 to 39 years, while the proportion of AIDS cases in children remains low (29 cases). The primary mode of transmission is by injecting drug use at 47 percent. Trends in the last three years may suggest a slight increase in sexual transmission, although it is unclear whether this is more a function of surveillance and reporting (Rhodes and others 2003). The incidence rate of AIDS and AIDS mortality decreased after HAART was introduced in 1997.

Sexually-transmitted Infections

Table 37 shows that there were 1,232 cases of syphilis reported in the 11 years

Table 37. Notifications of Syphilis by Sex 1992–2003

	No. of Notified Cases		
		Sex	
Year	Total	Men	Women
1992	55	33	22
1993	81	52	29
1994	98	62	36
1995	150	95	55
1996	130	83	47
1997	107	77	30
1998	87	52	35
1999	77	54	23
2000	75	43	32
2001	217	115	102
2002	78	48	30
2003	77	41	36
Total	**1,232**	**755**	**477**

Source: IPH Serbia 2004.

between 1992 and 2003. An increase during the mid-1990s was followed by a decrease and stabilization. The exception is an epidemic outbreak in 2001 in a closed center for persons with mental disability in Central Serbia when 150 residents contracted syphilis. The notification rate was around 1 per 100,000 in 2003. The trend of syphilis for men and women is similar. Changes in the trend, however, were more pronounced among men than among women, resulting in a noticeable decrease in the male to female ratio: from 1.9:1 in the 1995–1997 to 1.3 in the 2000–2002 period.

Gonorrhea is the second most frequently reported STI in Serbia, after chlamydia. Notifications between 1992 and 2003 are shown in Table 38. Since 1992, 5,213 cases of gonorrhea have been reported. The notification rate, at its peak in 1993, was 9.9 per 100,000 (16.2 for men and 3.7 for women), while in 2003, the rate was 1.5 per 100,000. The overall ratio of men to women was almost 3:1. Geographically, the highest notification rate in 2002 was recorded in Belgrade, 4.2 per 100,000 population.

Table 38. Notifications of Gonorrhea by Sex, 1992–2003

	No. of Notified Cases		
		Sex	
Year	Total	Men	Women
1992	759	640	119
1993	970	788	182
1994	838	671	167
1995	641	522	119
1996	398	303	95
1997	389	301	88
1998	239	176	63
1999	233	187	46
2000	247	193	54
2001	234	177	57
2002	153	131	22
2003	112	83	29
Total	5,213	4,172	1,041

Source: IPH Serbia 2004.

Figure 17. Acute Hepatitis C Infection by Age Groups, 1995–2002

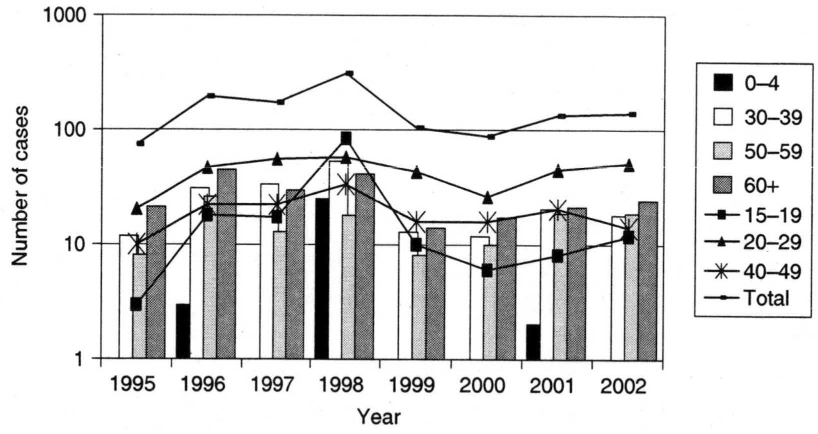

Source: IPH Serbia 2003.

Numbers and rates of notification of genital chlamydia infections largely depend on availability of the test kits; analysis of trends is not possible. A recent survey carried out among sexually active female adolescents in Belgrade found that every third adolescent interviewed had a genital chlamydia infection (Sedlecki 1999).

The reported incidence of Hepatitis C infection in Serbia has increased in the most recent years, especially among those between 20 to 29 years of age, indicating a strong suspicion of widespread needle sharing. In 2003, there were 148 cases reported. Men are more commonly infected (2:1), but there is no firm evidence to confirm a high prevalence rate among IDUs in Serbia (Rhodes and others 2003).

Vulnerability to HIV/AIDS: Contextual Factors

The population of Serbia and Montenegro in 2003 was 8.15 million, growing at 0.2 percent annually. Approximately 52 percent of the population lives in urban areas, compared to 70 percent for the entire Southern European region (PRB 2003). Within Serbia and Montenegro, 63 percent of the population is Serbian, 16.5 percent Albanian, 5 percent Montenegrin, and 3.3 percent Hungarian. Approximately 65 percent of the population is Christian Orthodox, 19 percent Muslim, 4 percent Roman Catholic, and 1 percent Protestant (U.S. Department of State 2003c).

In April 1992, the Federal Republic of Yugoslavia (FRY) was formed as the self-proclaimed successor to the Socialist Federal Republic of Yugoslavia. In February 2003, the FRY Parliament adopted a new constitutional charter establishing the Federal Union of Serbia and Montenegro, comprising the Republic of Serbia and the Republic of Montenegro. Under the provisions of the new constitutional charter, Serbia and Montenegro have some joint institutions, including the Presidency, Parliament, and a Council of Ministers, but operate separate economic, fiscal, monetary, and customs policies.

Between 1991 and 1999, FRY suffered severe economic decline, due to external as well as domestic factors. The decade of decline left a collapsed economy, fragile institution, and increased vulnerability. In 1993, hyperinflation was acute, and one of the severest worldwide. In 1999, GDP declined by 16 percent. By 2000, when the country began its transition to democracy and a market economy, GDP had fallen to less than half its 1989 level. In addition, the wars in Bosnia, Croatia, and Kosovo left Serbia and Montenegro with 450,000 refugees and 240,000 internally displaced persons, in addition to other economically and socially vulnerable groups (World Bank 2003e).

This scenario has led to an overall deterioration in the quality and availability of social services. Public health facilities and medical care have been undermined by reduced contributions to the national health insurance fund. Investments in education have been cut, with resultant declines in learning conditions and the quality of teaching. There have been numerous interruptions in schooling in recent years because of teacher strikes and bombing. Social welfare services have been reduced, including allowances for children living in poverty. Unemployment, insecurity, and stress have weakened parental care capacities. The steep fall in the standard of living has resulted in a deterioration of nutritional practices, especially among the poor.

Table 39. Vulnerability Factors—Serbia	
GNI per Capita World Bank. 2003	US$1,400
Unemployment Government. 2002	38.7%
Poverty World Bank. 2003	11% below poverty line
Mobility Serbia and Montenegro Rhodes et. al. 2003	▨ >500,000 displaced people ▨ 242,000 IDPs ▨ 389,000 refugees
Trafficking	Anti trafficking efforts poorly organized MSM and women working in tourism industry are particularly vulnerable groups

Economy

Serbia is a lower middle-income country with GNI per capita of US$ 1,400. Serbia experienced a sharp contraction of GDP per capita in the 1990s, from approximately $ 2,450 per capita in 1990 to an estimated $ 900 per capita 10 years later. However, after a delayed transition, the country appears to be progressing toward a market economy despite the political turmoil of the past two years. The economy grew at 5.5 percent in 2001 and 4 percent in 2002, although growth is now slowing (World Bank 2003e). In July 2001, a US$4 billion, four-year comprehensive economic recovery and transition program was supported at a Donors' Conference in Brussels, co-organized by the World Bank and the European Commission.

Poverty

Poverty rose sharply in the 1990s and remains widespread. Using a poverty threshold level of €2.40 a day finds that 11 percent of the Serbian population falls below the poverty line. Those most vulnerable to poverty include households with unemployed heads, single parents, the elderly, school-age children, large families (with three or more children), rural populations, people with low educational levels, Roma, refugees, and displaced persons, all of whom are concurrently vulnerable to acquiring HIV and being able to access HIV/AIDS care and support services.

Serbia's 2002 Survey on the Living Standard of the Population showed that among individuals below the poverty line, 30 percent have a diagnosed chronic medical condition, in comparison with 27 percent percent above the poverty line. Approximately 17 percent of all adults in Serbia can be considered "education poor." Health poverty affects between 4–6 percent of the population in Serbia and Montenegro; many poor cannot afford medical treatment and have low utilization rates. Certain regions are poorer than others. Moreover, there is often a disparity in poverty levels within regions (World Bank 2003h).

In 2003, the Government prepared a Poverty Reduction Strategy (PRSP) with the support of the Bank, UNDP, multi-bi external assistance and in cooperation with the civil society. The Interim PRSP does not put emphasis on public health and prevention despite growing problems in health status and access, and lack of funding for preventive services. With regard to related expenditure, the PRSP is vague, stating that, "The implementation of other programs should be phased in according to availability of resources, including those freed up by efficiency savings from other areas of the health sector" (Government of Serbia 2003).

Mobility

Serbia, as other countries in Southeast Europe, has a highly mobile population. It is estimated that over half a million refugees and IDPs live in poverty. In 2003, there were 389,000 refugees and over 242,000 Internally Displaced Persons (IDPs) in Serbia and Montenegro. According to the Serbian Commission on Refugees, there are approximately 13,000 refugees living in collective centers (refugee camps), and almost 10,000 IDPs in camps. There are many more refugees and IDPs living outside of the camps, independently or with local relatives, but refugees and IDPs in collective settlements are often considered the most vulnerable (Rhodes 2003).

UNICEF's MICS[11] indicated that child refugees and internally displaced children who are living in collective accommodation centers have poorer health and nutritional status than children among the general population, and receive less schooling. Those living in collective centers suffer in particular because the state has been unable to deliver social services in general and these groups do not have the resources to seek out private alternatives. To date, no systematic governmental strategies have been developed for working with displaced populations, although there are several NGOs working in this sector. Private medical practices have flourished in recent years but are expensive in comparison to the public health services and unaffordable to refugees and IDPs (Rhodes and others 2003).

Travel to other countries has been restricted due to UN imposed economic sanctions and national visa entry restrictions, but nonetheless, many people are working abroad and traveling to Europe. Although providing needed economic opportunities, the transport and tourism sectors entail increases in mobility, possible regroupings of family units, and exposure to new sexual networks, which may have significant ramifications for HIV transmission. To date, no systematic strategies for HIV/AIDS have been developed for these populations, and the experience of other countries indicates they are vulnerable to HIV infection.

Vulnerable Groups

Vulnerable groups in Serbia face increasing risk due to the impact of the conflict, poverty and high unemployment, oppressive and isolationist government policies, deteriorating

---

11. Multiple Indicator Cluster Survey II (UNICEF 2001). The MICS interviewed women and children from 5,731 households.

economic conditions, a decline in the provision of basic services, and a breakdown of societal and cultural norms. These factors have resulted in the presence of increased risk behavior among young people, particularly those between 15 to 24 years.

Youth. Serbia's population is older than that of Albania and Macedonia. Approximately 20 percent of the population is under age 15. In 2000, the country's median age was 35 (UN 2003). Some of the key findings of UNICEF's RAR[12] show that Serbia's youth often have incomplete knowledge about STIs and HIV/AIDS and lack the life skills necessary to avoid infection. The RAR found that young people engage in risky sexual behavior. They often have more than one partner and have sex while under the influence of one or more substances. Even when young people are aware of condoms as a prevention measure for STIs and HIV/AIDS, they fail to use them on a regular basis.

The 2000 MICS found that there are serious disparities with regard to the educational coverage of some children, including those from specific ethnic groups such as Roma and Vlahs; those with special needs; those from villages in underdeveloped regions; and children from IDP families (UNICEF 2003a).

Existing health and social services are not youth-friendly and young people reported that they do not obtain information and life skills about sexual health and related issues from either their parents or the formal education system. Peers and older siblings are relied upon as a source of information, rather than parents and teachers. UNICEF also reports that few efforts are being undertaken to develop formal curricula in schools to include education on substance abuse, sex education, and condom promotion. Young people are not part of the dialogue on critical issues such as HIV/AIDS, healthy lifestyles, and have few mechanisms for participation in decisions that affect their lives.

Sex Workers and Trafficking. In the absence of scientific data estimating the size of commercial sex worker populations, most estimates are wide ranging and rely on anecdotal reports. A newspaper[13] estimated 3,000 sex workers in Belgrade in early 2002, indicating that approximately 50 percent was registered by the police. The City of Belgrade Department for Public Order and Peace at the Ministry of Internal Affairs undertakes regular raids among female CSWs in Belgrade, collecting data on the number of sex workers against whom charges were made. These data, which provide a partial picture on trends in sex work in the capital, show that in the last two and a half years, almost 700 CSWs have been detained, with 74 percent of them street sex workers. There has been an unprecedented increase in the number of CSWs identified and detained in the last 18 months, especially within the first six months of 2003, when almost as many were detained as in the whole of 2002 (around 230; Rhodes and others 2003).

---

12. UNICEF's Rapid Assessment (2002a). Field work for this study was undertaken between October 2001 and January 2002. In Serbia, questionnaires were administered to 464 drug users and injecting drug users, 299 young MSM, and 116 sex workers. Interviews were conducted with 142 drug users/injecting drug users and a total of 147 drug users/injecting drug users participated in 16 focus groups. Interviews were also conducted with 94 young MSM and a total of 100 young MSM participated in 25 focus groups. Interviews were conducted with 25 sex workers and a total of 36 sex workers participated in focus groups.

13. Nedeljni Telegraf (February 20, 2002).

Most CSWs interviewed for the UNICEF RAR stated they would like STI and HIV testing to be more accessible. Among other findings, the RAR showed that Roma sex workers, unaware of risk behaviors, often agree to have sex without condoms if their clients are willing to pay more for it. However, sex workers who are aware of risk behaviors and are working to support their families use condoms most of the time (Wong 2002c). The mean age of CSWs was 21 years and 57 percent used drugs. Overall, 76 percent thought that they were at risk of HIV or other STIs, and 51 percent had been tested for HIV. Of those who injected drugs, 85 percent shared drug-injecting equipment and 99 percent had sex under the influence of drugs. Approximately 60 percent reported that they always used condoms during sex.

Although there are no reliable data on the extent of women trafficked or exhibiting risk behavior among trafficked women, experts view trafficked sex workers as an especially vulnerable group whose human and citizenship rights are highly compromised. Evidence suggests that Belgrade has been a major transit center for trafficked women over the past 10 to 15 years, with women sold and bought in Belgrade on their way to Bosnia and Herzegovina or Western Europe. The increased intensity of police raids is said to have shifted transit and trafficking routes from the cities into the suburbs. Two other sex work populations were also highlighted in terms of their vulnerability. The first was transvestites, who were described as being usually full-time sex workers, belonging to the lowest economic classes, and who are often of Muslim background and often refugees or IDPs. The second group was sex workers who worked in connection with the tourist industry (Rhodes and others 2003).

According to the U.S. Department of State (2003), the Government of Serbia and Montenegro does not fully comply with the minimum standards for the elimination of trafficking. During 2002, the federal and republic governments increased their capacity to protect victims and to cooperate with NGOs. However, lack of proper treatment of victims in court, low court convictions, and potential government complicity are still serious weaknesses in the government's ability to meet the minimum standards. Data on Serbia's response to trafficking, including detail on governmental, donor, and NGO interventions, have been compiled online by the South East European Regional Initiative against Human Trafficking, funded by UNICEF, OSCE, and UNHCHR. In particular, female and young refugees and IDPs are reportedly at risk for sexual abuse. For example, female refugees crossing the border looking for work who stay with relatives may be at risk of sexual abuse by these relatives. Because of the cramped living conditions in the camps, children are considered to be at risk for sexual abuse by their parents or guardians and this may well affect both girls and boys (Rhodes and others 2003).

MSM. Most MSM interviewed by RAR considered that they were stigmatized by society and can sense various degrees of homophobia. Many have serious doubts about the anonymity of HIV testing. Of these, 76 percent thought that they were at risk of HIV or other STIs, and 41 percent had been tested for HIV. The mean age at first sexual intercourse was 16.5 years, and 38 percent had between 2 and 5 sexual partners in the past year; 19 percent had between 6 and 10 sexual partners in the past year; and 8 percent percent had more than 10 sexual partners in the past year. Almost two-thirds (61 percent) always used condoms during sex.

Since 1994, homosexuality is no longer been punishable by law in Serbia, and not a single case of prosecution has been recorded. However, a high level of stigmatization and prejudice persists towards MSM. Consequently, MSM remain largely underground. There was a consensus among those interviewed that MSM comprise one of the priority vulnerable populations for HIV prevention in Serbia and Montenegro. The DFID HIV Prevention Among Vulnerable Populations Initiative in Serbia and Montenegro (Rhodes and others 2003) identified three main vulnerable populations of MSM: young men (especially underage boys), MSM involved in sex work (which is illegal), and bisexual men (in particular men who define themselves as heterosexual but who have sex with other men). (This latter group may be less likely to be informed than most gay men).

Drug Users. Estimates of drug users in the early 1990s ranged from 13,000 to 30,000 people, with 20,000 users in Belgrade alone. The current estimate is roughly around 100,000. While the Belgrade Institute for Public Health has maintained a register of drug addicts for the city of Belgrade since 1980, data do not distinguish injecting from non-injecting drug users. The only available estimate suggests that 15 percent of registered drug users are injectors.

The mean age when they first began injected drugs was 18.2 years. Almost all (98 percent) had had sexual intercourse, and 82 percent thought that they were at risk of HIV or other STIs. Over half (57 percent) had been tested for HIV, and shared drug-injecting equipment. Over half (51 percent) had between 2 and 5 sexual partners in the past year; only 15 percent always used condoms during sex; and 14 percent had sex in return for money or drugs (Wong 2002c.)

Among drugs users not injecting drugs, most RAR respondents reported feeling stigmatized and rejected by society, family, friends, and by the health care system that is

---

Table 40. Knowledge, Attitudes, and Practices—Serbia

IDUs	▓ 62% do not consider drug use to be risk factor
	▓ 57% share needles
	▓ 95% have sex
	▓ 30% never use condoms
CSW	▓ 57% used drugs
	▓ 99% had sex while on drugs
	▓ 85% IDUs shared injecting equipment
	▓ 60% report use of condoms
	▓ Paid more if not using condoms
	▓ 51% tested for HIV
MSM	▓ HIV prevalence rate 2.3%
	▓ 77% use drugs
	▓ 38% have 2–5 sex partners per year
	▓ 19% have more than 6 sex partners per year
	▓ 61% always use condoms
	▓ 41% tested for HIV

expected to provide them with treatment and care. Over 50 percent of the participants had engaged in crime to gain money for drugs, and participants reported that medical staff often treated them as law offenders. Over 33 percent had experienced drug overdoses. Almost all (95 percent) had had sexual intercourse, and 34 percent had been tested for HIV. Of those who had sexual intercourse, 42 percent percent had between two and five sexual partners in the past year, and 24 percent percent always used condoms during sex; 13 percent percent had sex in return for money or drugs (Wong 2002c).

According to UN Office of Drugs and Crime (2003), cocaine consumption in Serbia and Montenegro has been increasing. Heroin seizures increased dramatically, from 15,425 kilograms in 1997 to 62,518 kilograms in 2001. However, this scenario could be due to improved reporting, law enforcement efforts, or an increase in trafficking. Trends in seizures of cocaine, cannabis, amphetamine-type stimulants, and hallucinogens are impeded by lack of reporting data.

Early and occasional reports of injecting drug use appeared in major cities of Serbia during the mid- to late-1970s, with heroin use becoming an established problem in the early 1980s, being most prevalent in Belgrade. Throughout the 1990s, heroin use and injecting has diffused outwards from the capital to other major cities in Serbia, including Kragujevac, Novi Sad, and Nis. Studies are needed to estimate the size of the drug injecting populations.

The sharing of used injection equipment is said to play a significant role in the spread of HIV as well as Hepatitis B and C. In one recent study, as many as 43 percent of IDUs reported injecting with used equipment, while in recent RAR studies 57 percent of IDUs reported recent needle and syringe sharing. Studies also suggest that a significant number of IDUs report multiple sexual partners, with one study indicating that 32 percent reported between two and five sexual partners in the previous year, and 21 percent reporting more than five partners. In combination with relatively high rates of multiple partners, evidence indicates that consistent condom use is rare, with one study showing that a third of IDUs never use condoms. Estimates also suggest an overlap between drug injecting and sex work among female IDUs (Rhodes and others 2003).

The extent of first treatment demand among heroin users at the Institute for Dependence Diseases in Belgrade is estimated to have increased three to four times over recent years to some 1,000 new clients seeking treatment per year. Experts indicated that it is important to recognize that there is an average of six years elapsing between heroin initiation and demand for first treatment, and that according to a survey conducted in 1992, every injector in treatment knew of between 10 to 20 other IDUs who were not in contact with treatment services. It is almost certainly the case that the majority of IDUs remain out of contact with treatment services (Rhodes and others 2003).

In general terms, Serbians who inject drugs are socially and economically vulnerable. The majority of IDUs (over 60 percent in one study) are unemployed, almost 10 percent are thought to have participated in the recent 1992–1994 war, and 25 percent have been prisoners. Everyday risk management from the perspective of drug injectors is also closely associated with avoidance of arrest or detainment.

The Basic Criminal Code links drug possession with a sentence of a fine or imprisonment of up to three years; drug production or dealing with at least five years imprisonment; organization or being part of production or dealing networks with imprisonment of at least seven years; and possessing or providing drug production equipment or materials with imprisonment with six months to five years. Of greater concern in the context of harm reduction and HIV prevention initiatives are laws relating to the facilitation of drug use, especially groups of people, potentially linked with at least three years imprisonment, with persons said to encourage another to engage in illicit drug use punishable by one to five years imprisonment. While these laws do not technically prevent or disrupt the development or expansion of harm reduction services, including syringe distribution, a perception of reticence or concern may, nonetheless, slow their implementation (Rhodes and others 2003).

Prisoners. Although some recent estimates have put HIV prevalence within Serbian prisons as low as 1 percent, others suggest HIV prevalence around 10 percent. To date no systematic assessment of the prevalence of HIV has been carried out in Serbian (or Montenegrin) prisons. Overcrowding, in particular, is a common problem in prisons, and has become more intense during and after the State of Emergency following the assassination of Prime Minister Djindjic, which saw large numbers of people, especially drug users, detained. In some cases, capacity is exceeded more than twofold. Generally, there are limited resources for HIV testing within the prison system, and consequently, no routine HIV testing service (Rhodes and others 2003).

In 2002, the Organization for Security and Cooperation in Europe carried out an assessment of the quality of prison services in Belgrade, identifying a number of shortcomings, many of which were common to the penitentiary system in Serbia as a whole. The Central Prison Hospital was found to violate European and international standards, including the UN standard Minimum Rules for the Treatment of Prisoners, which stipulates that material and moral conditions ensure respect for human dignity. Other shortcomings related to the lack of rehabilitation activities, limited professional staff training, and the need for extensive refurbishment "to stop enduring terrible physical conditions by prisoners and the staff" (Rhodes and others 2003).

Roma. According to official estimates, there are 107,000 Roma in Serbia, but independent estimates suggest this number may be as high as 500,000. Many Roma in Serbia are refugees or IDPs resulting from the many regional conflicts over the past decade. The majority of IDPs, and most likely unregistered Roma IDPs, are scattered around the surrounding areas of large cities. Some 16,000 Roma IDPs live in official or unofficial collective centers, reportedly in very poor conditions. This is over 40 percent of the officially registered Roma IDP population. There is a general consensus that Roma IDPs form one of the most vulnerable populations, having little or no access to public health, education, or social welfare services, and suffering considerable levels of discrimination and stigmatization. According to international agency representatives with whom the DFID HIV Prevention Among Populations Initiative in Serbia and Montenegro met in July 2003, the disenfranchised status of the Roma put them at increased risk of HIV and other infectious diseases (Rhodes and others 2003).

HIV/AIDS Awareness and Knowledge

UNICEF's MICS found that, in general, adolescents were less informed than adults about HIV/AIDS. Although the 60 percent believed that using a condom every time can prevent

HIV transmission, significantly fewer adolescents believed that having only one uninfected sex partner can prevent HIV transmission (55 percent). Approximately 25 percent of adolescents agreed that abstaining from sex prevents HIV transmission. Finally, just 16 percent were aware of all three ways to contract HIV and 73 percent were aware of at least one means (UNICEF 2001). Adolescent women (aged 15–19) were the least likely of any age group to have been tested and the least likely to know the result. Finally, women with no education or only primary education were less likely than women with more education to be tested and least likely to have been told the result of the test.

Overall, 63 percent of women knew that a healthy looking person can be infected with HIV, yet only 38 percent knew AIDS cannot be transmitted by mosquito bites. Slightly less than one in three women knew all three modes of transmission. Women in rural areas were less likely to identify both misconceptions about AIDS transmission than urban women. Women with higher education were more likely to recognize both misconceptions (51 percent) than women with secondary (32 percent) and primary or no education (22 percent). Approximately 61 percent of women knew that HIV/AIDS can be transmitted from mother to child; about 65 percent said that transmission was possible during pregnancy; 51 percent said that transmission was possible at delivery; and only 37 percent agreed that AIDS could be transmitted through breast milk. Knowledge that AIDS could be transmitted from mother to child was higher in urban (66 percent) than rural areas (55 percent); it was also higher among more-educated women (76 percent among women with higher education, versus 50 percent among women with no education or only primary education).

The 2000 MICS found that 45 percent of women of reproductive age knew a place to get tested for AIDS. Women living in Belgrade were most likely to know a place (61 percent), followed by Central Serbia (excluding Belgrade) (42 percent), and Vojvodina (41 percent). Only 27 percent of women with primary education or no education knew of a place to get tested compared to 47 percent of women with secondary and 67 percent with higher education. About 6 percent of women have been tested for AIDS. The vast majority of women who have been tested were told the results (85 percent).

The survey provided information about discriminatory attitudes as well. Approximately 29 percent of women aged 15–49 agreed with at least one discriminatory statement toward people with HIV/AIDS. One of four respondents overall believed that a teacher with HIV/AIDS should not be allowed to work. Urban women and those with secondary or higher education were more likely to express this discriminatory attitude than rural women and those with no education or only primary education. Approximately 17 percent of women would not buy food from a person with HIV/AIDS. These results may be related to greater awareness of HIV/AIDS (although insufficient knowledge), among urban women and those who are more educated.

Health Care in Serbia

Under the 2003 constitutional charter, the former federal ministry of health, which had a relatively limited regulatory role, has been abolished and its functions delegated to the republican level. The health system is characterized by an extensive network of public facilities, from the ambulantas (the health stations that are scattered throughout the country) to the clinical centers (tertiary university hospitals located in Belgrade, Nis, and Novi Sad).

Although the level of service inputs (staff numbers, infrastructure) is almost identical to that which was operating in 1990, the financial resources flowing into the sector have significantly declined. The fall in resources led to cuts in non-salary operating costs, capital maintenance, repairs and replacement, and reduction in the real value of salaries. Only one-third of hospitals in Serbia have functioning sterilization systems. Approximately 75 percent of the medical equipment in health facilities is over 10 years old. With support from the World Bank, the Government of Serbia is preparing a Health Sector Human Resources Strategy.

The Government has identified a number of immediate priorities, including the reform of health financing, with procedures to improve the effectiveness and efficiency of the contracting process, including private sector participation. Other priorities include improved access to drugs and replacing medical equipment. In 2003, the Ministry of Health in Serbia prepared a draft Health Strategy for 2003–2015. The draft includes specific short-, medium-, and long-term goals for the reform of the health sector and proposes a number of changes to health financing, essential health packages, and the mandates of Serbian health institutions (Stevenson 2003).

The Institutes of Public Health (a network that comprises the Republican Center Batut and 23 regional IPHs) and the Sanitary Inspection Service provide public health functions in Serbia. The health centers provide extensive public health services, although many functions in this structure are not explicitly targeted at public health, and financing of these services is unclear. The main source of income for the IPH is the HIF, which reimburses the institutes for testing and other services. Furthermore, the IPHs receive transfers from the Government to implement the 50 official public health programs and perform activities in disease control, monitoring, and surveillance. In terms of employment, about 10 percent of the total health care workforce is engaged in public health functions. The private health sector started to develop more than 10 years ago but has not been incorporated into the data for the republican health system or health insurance.

Funding of Health Services

The Serbia health system is financed through a combination of public finance and private contributions. The two main sources of public funding are the central Government budget and the Health Insurance Fund. Contributions to the Health Insurance Fund are raised through a payroll tax of about 15 percent on salaries and wages. Approximately 92 percent of the population is covered by the compulsory health insurance. Funds for health care for the uninsured part of the population are provided through the Government budget. The Government guarantees universal access to a liberal package of health services. Yet, it lacks necessary incentives for efficient utilization of resources, delivers poor quality health care, and relies heavily on formal and informal out-of-pocket payments.

As noted by World Bank (2002e), a comprehensive analysis of Serbia's financial situation of the health sector is difficult. Data on health care financing is scarce, and, if it does exist, is often inconsistent. It is estimated that public health expenditure in Serbia was about 9 percent of GDP in 1998. This percentage decreased to slightly less than 7 percent in the years thereafter, and is estimated to have been relatively stable at this level in 2000 and 2001. Private health expenditure is estimated to amount to around 2 percent of GDP.

In terms of total health expenditure, this places Serbia with around 10 percent of GDP, at the higher end of Central and Eastern European countries and close to the expenditure levels in many Western European countries. However, in terms of per capita funding, the absolute amounts are very low, ranging from US$67 to $107 per capita, according to population estimates. The budget of the Ministry of Health (excluding HIF revenues) accounted for 1.8 percent of the state budget in 2002. Despite shrinking overall Government revenues, there has been some success in lobbying for a budget increase for health care recently, and this figure increased to 3.7 percent in 2002.

Funding for HIV/AIDS

Currently Serbia has no direct HIV/AIDS related allocations in its national budget. However, in 2002, $5.7 million was spent on HIV/AIDS. Of this, $3.9 million for treatment expenses was covered by the health insurance budget; the remaining $1.7 million, comprising $0.2 million for prevention and $1.5 million for testing/screening, was covered by external assistance.

Serbia plans to fund preparation of an HIV/AIDS strategic plan with funding from the GFATM Knowledge, Attitudes, and Practices—Serbia. In Round 1 of the GFATM, Serbia's HIV/AIDS proposal was approved for $2.7 million over two years. A grant agreement was signed in April 2003, and as of the end of 2003, $1 million had been disbursed.

At present, around 500 AIDS patients in Serbia receive regular check-ups at the Clinic of Infectious Diseases in Belgrade. Of those patients, around 300 are on antiretroviral treatment (ARV). This treatment is covered through HIF and MOH sources, and Serbia is the only one of the countries studied that finances ARV treatment publicly. Costs for ARV treatment in Serbia amount to approximately $15,000 per patient per year, adding up to an estimated total of $4.5 million per year. For regular monitoring and testing of AIDS patients, another $450 per patient would be required, adding a total of around $225,000 per year to the treatment costs. Due to financial restrictions and scarcity of test kits and supplies, only about half of the required tests are done at present, at a total cost of around $120,000. In addition, the HIF pays around $4 million per year for testing of blood donations.

There is a huge potential for savings on ARV drugs in Serbia. However, no attempts to reduce the costs of drug procurement have taken place. Procurement of ARV drugs is not well planned, and the financial situation of the HIF only allows for limited orders at a time, thus weakening the leverage of the Government. Taking into account prices negotiated by neighboring countries, it is estimated that the costs for ARV treatment could be reduced to half the current price, that is, around $7,500 per patient per year, with a cumulative savings potential of around $2.2 million. The Clinical Centre in Belgrade, with three specialized doctors and one clinical psychologist, is the only site for HIV/AIDS therapy in Serbia. This means that patients from outside Belgrade, currently around 33 percent of all patients, face considerable travel and opportunity costs for receiving treatment.

Estimated Resource Needs for HIV/AIDS

A recent study of the World Bank and UNAIDS (2003) has estimated the total funding requirements to effectively combat HIV/AIDS in Serbia until 2007 (Table 41). These estimates

Table 41. Estimated Resource Needs and Funding Gaps for HIV/AIDS Treatment, Serbia					
	2003 $000	2004 $000	2005 $000	2006 $000	2007 $000
Total expenditure on HIV/AIDS (1)	5,700	5,700	5,700	5,700	5,700
GFATM Grant (1)		1,135	1,584	544	313
Estimated HIV/AIDS Funding Required for Serbia & Montenegro (2)	19,738	20,570	21,097	20,168	16,470
Total funding gap (Serbia)	14,038	13,735	13,813	13,924	10,457

Source: 1. GFATM proposal, 2. World Band and UNAIDS estimates.

cover resource needs for comprehensive care (including ARV) and prevention programs. Taking into account these estimates, there was a cumulative resource gap of more than $13.4 million in 2002. In per capita terms, this translates into an approximate funding need in the range of US$1.80 per person per year, or between 1.7 to 2.7 percent of the total current per capita spending on health. In the years to come, this resource gap is likely to widen until 2006, if no additional resources can be mobilized, and will result in a funding gap of approximately $1.30 per capita over the next four years, before declining to slightly less than $1 per capita in 2007. These estimates point at the urgent need to mobilize additional resources for the prevention and treatment of HIV/AIDS. By doing this, effective prevention and treatment procedures that lower the burden of disease stemming from HIV/AIDS infections could be provided with a relatively moderate increase in health expenditure.

The already existing funding gap is particularly severe for some special institutions with high-risk groups for HIV. For example, the Central Prison Hospital in Belgrade reported that, of the resource needs of approximately 4 million Serbian Dinars (approximately $70,000) per month, only half of the amount is approved in the budget, and only half of the budgeted amount (one-quarter of the resource needs) is indeed available and will be disbursed to the facility. As a consequence, no HIV/AIDS treatment can be provided in the prison, and the institution has accumulated substantial arrears for drugs and supplies.

Government and Civil Society Action on HIV/AIDS

Strategic, Policy, and Regulatory Framework

The new country leadership is aware of the need for urgent renewal of national efforts in HIV/AIDS prevention. In 2001, Serbia established the Republic National AIDS Committee (RAC). The RAC function in close cooperation with the UN Theme Group for HIV/AIDS and brings together representatives of other international organizations and a number of national actors from different sectors and from all levels. The RAC functions as the national Country Coordination Mechanism for Global Fund related matters. It is also working on

Table 42. Government Intervention and Institutional Arrangements—Serbia

Intersectoral coordination	▨ Country Coordination Mechanism established to request GFATM grant
National HIV/AIDS Strategy and Legislation	▨ Controlling HIV/AIDS in Serbia: A Comprehensive Country Strategic and an Emergency Action Plan ▨ GFATM application approved
Government institution responsible for HIV/AIDS	▨ Republican AIDS Commission undertakes strategic planning process Institute for Public Health, Belgrade ▨ Responsible for collecting and analyzing epidemiological data ▨ HIV testing (also available at regional IPHs) ▨ Some pre- and posttest counseling (Belgrade only) ▨ HIV test confirmation (Belgrade only)

a joint framework for an overall state policy and intervention in the field of HIV/AIDS, in cooperation with civil society and the private sector. By the end of 2003, the RAC had prepared the Republican Strategy for HIV/AIDS. Establishment of the RAC is a significant step forward, particularly in an effort to broaden the strategies for HIV/AIDS beyond the health sector. The RAC also provides support to the relatively new and growing NGO sector in their efforts to control the epidemic.

The only two official state documents regulating HIV/AIDS concerns have their origins in the former Yugoslavia, dating from 1986 and 1988. The Program and Regulation on Health Protection of Infectious Diseases in Serbia, 2002–2010, mentions goals and measures for reducing the AIDS incidence and mortality, and also stresses the importance of reducing the incidence rate of gonorrhea, syphilis, and chlamydia.

Among the next steps for improving the national AIDS strategy, the following goals were identified: decentralization of national AIDS programs and mobilization of district and municipal level authorities; formulation of national strategic AIDS plans, as well as local level strategies, with active civil society and local level participation; strategies to address factors that make individuals particularly vulnerable to HIV infection, including economic insecurity, poverty, lack of empowerment of women, lack of education, and discrimination. Currently, there is no specific legal framework to protect the rights of PLWHA. UNHCHR and the UN Theme Group on HIV/AIDS are examining legal frameworks to incorporate a human rights approach (IOM and UNICEF 2002).

Serbia's Country Coordinating Mechanism comprises numerous ministry representatives, NGOs, and multinational groups. The approved HIV/AIDS GFATM proposal (GFATM 2003b) comprises six components that address current problems in areas relevant to the implementation of the AIDS Program, including:

▨ Development of a national HIV strategy;
▨ Education of health care staff;
▨ HIV education in schools;

- Social marketing of condoms;
- PMTCT, including access to antiretroviral therapy for HIV-positive mothers and their infants; and
- HIV prevention among high-risk groups with special focus on IDUs, commercial sex workers, and MSM.

HIV/AIDS and STIs Surveillance

According to the Rapid Assessment of Serbia HIV/AIDS/STI Surveillance System, Serbia has a well-established public health and clinical care infrastructure. However, there are considerable problems in reporting and surveillance of HIV. Further, surveillance is passive and there is no systematic active or sentinel surveillance in place. Testing and reporting is particularly problematic for rural areas and regions outside of Belgrade.

The public health surveillance network in Serbia comprises 22 district Institutes of Public Health, each of which is responsible for notifications of communicable diseases to the Republican Institute of Public Health in Belgrade. The Republican Institute of Public Health has a national statutory responsibility for the prevention and surveillance of 70 notifiable infectious diseases. The private health sector started to develop more than 10 years ago, but its data has not been incorporated into the health system or health insurance. Recently, a draft of a protocol for HIV/AIDS and STI surveillance in Serbia, as well as for other infectious diseases, has been delivered to all IPHs and other relevant institutions, including the members of Republican Infectious Diseases Commission, for adoption and implementation.

Reporting of infectious diseases is regulated by the acts set out in the Federal and Republic Official Gazettes. Current relevant law regulations include: Law on Health Protection of Infectious Diseases; Reporting Infectious Diseases Acts; and Regulation on Health Protection of Infectious Diseases. Generally, the work of epidemiologists is carried out in isolation from other disciplines. For example, the Republic Institute for Public Health has no communication with the Clinics and Institutes of Dermatology and Venerology, which are responsible for STI treatment. Although new Government plans and programs are now addressing these shortcomings, there remains insufficient dissemination of analysis to reporting sources. Thus, surveillance data have not been optimally utilized to target prevention and control activities.

The number of persons tested for HIV is very low (1.5 HIV tested per 1,000 population, excluding voluntary blood donors). Testing availability varies across Serbia. All donated blood is screened free of charge at transfusion centers. Within Serbia, testing is available in both the public and the private laboratory system. Free HIV testing is limited, but is reported to be free for everyone around the time of World AIDS Day; it is also free for students at the Belgrade University Institute for Student Health, and for high-risk pregnant women. Patients with active TB or STIs are not routinely tested for HIV. Pre- and post-test counseling is limited. HIV is tested by ELISA and confirmed at the HIV/AIDS Center in Belgrade by a third ELISA and Western Blot (WB) before the result is registered as confirmed. The number of people who do not report for confirmation testing is unknown. Western Blot is also available at the Belgrade Institute of Public Health, at the Students' Institute of Public Health, and at some private laboratories.

Table 43. Government Intervention and Institutional Arrangements—Serbia	
Testing	▓ ELISA testing is available in several transfusion centers
	▓ Positive samples are sent to central laboratories in Belgrade for Western Blot
	▓ Testing rate is very low (1.5 per 1,000)
	▓ Free testing available for some groups (students of Belgrade University, high risk pregnant women); and during World AIDS Day Campaign
Surveillance	▓ TB patients and patients with STI are not routinely screened
	▓ 22 district IPHs report to the Republican Institute of Public Health in Belgrade.
HIV/AIDS Notification	▓ Notification is done at cantonal levels using preprinted report form
Blood Safety	▓ All donated blood screened free of charge
	▓ Free testing for HIV is offered to all blood donors
Prevention	▓ Preventive activities are undertaken mostly by NGOs
Treatment	▓ Treatment provided to 500 AIDS patients including 300 on ARVs at the AIDS Clinic at the Clinic for Infectious and Tropical Diseases in Belgrade
	▓ ARV costs 1,000$ a month

Laboratory tests for STI diagnosis are not available on a regular basis. Specialist treatment continues to rely on laboratory diagnoses of STIs, but given the shortage of diagnostic tests, it is likely that considerable syndromic management, with or without WHO guidelines, is done in Serbia. The availability of drugs for STI treatment is also uncertain.

HIV/AIDS and STIs Prevention and Control in the Public System

Youth-friendly counseling and services, particularly in the area of reproductive health, do not exist in Serbia, except in Belgrade. Of those services that do exist, most programs focus on HIV/AIDS and some include programs on STIs. One program largely devoted to STIs is "Promoting Reproductive Health of Adolescents," implemented by the Republican Center for Family Planning at the Institute for Mother and Child, Belgrade. One of its activities, during 1999 and 2000, was the development of a model counseling service for reproductive health for young people. Directed at the primary health care level, the model includes educational and promotional activities in the area of diagnosing and treating reproductive health disorders among adolescents. It was funded by the Ministry for Family Care, UNICEF, and UNAIDS.

Although some peer education and educational life skills programs exist, they are not systematically implemented (IOM and UNICEF 2002). Sexual health is not part of the compulsory school program. This is expected to be rectified in the next two years by the implementation of the GFATM grant. The Ministry of Education is engaged in a global reform of the school curricula, training of teachers, introducing active learning and a more open education system, which also includes health education. UNICEF, UN Theme Group for AIDS, IPH, and RAC are assisting the Ministry of Education in designing the health education related to HIV/AIDS, STIs, and reproductive health. However, funding for education has been declining throughout the past decade and is now among the lowest in Europe.

HIV/AIDS, STIs, and Drug Use Treatment

At present, the HIV/AIDS Center, at the Institute for Infectious and Tropical Diseases, Clinical University Center in Belgrade, is the only provider of HIV treatment in Serbia and Montenegro. Approximately 500 patients are registered at the Center, about 25 percent of all registered HIV/AIDS cases. About 450 patients are on HAART. This treatment is covered through HIF and MOH sources. Twenty beds are available, which is clearly insufficient. Simple or routine blood tests frequently cannot be carried out due to equipment failure. Furthermore, there is inadequate funding to cover the costs of monitoring patients' health status and disease progression (for example, CD4 counts). The average expected survival of PLWHA that receive treatment at the Center is said to be eight years. Although there is one project, supported by Norwegian Aid, which aims to develop home care and mobile teams of nurses, there is insufficient capacity to meet the demand for HIV treatment and care (Rhodes and others 2003).

The City Institute for Dermatology and Venereology is a center of excellence for STI diagnosis and management in Belgrade. Most STIs are diagnosed and treated there. More than 30 percent of STI diagnoses made in this clinic are of chlamydia infection. Patients come to the clinic in Belgrade from across the country where a consultation costs around 500 dinars or about €8 (the average monthly salary in Serbia is about €250). It is believed that a majority of STI patients may now be treated in the private sector. There are a few private clinics in Serbia and many patients use them because confidentiality is guaranteed. However, in the private sector diagnosis is often carried out without laboratory testing, cases are not reported, and partners will, generally, not be notified. Private doctors often use a syndromic approach to STI treatment and a consultation costs about 30 per visit. Laboratory tests in private laboratories cost from €12–25. Self-treatment is believed to be common with patients obtaining cheap over-the-counter antibiotics from pharmacies. It is believed that doses are often inadequate.

Medical treatment for drug withdrawal for IDUs is currently only available at the Institute for Drug Dependency. No methadone program is available and no alternative treatments exist. Some individuals go abroad for private treatment, which is very expensive and available for only a few individuals.

HIV/AIDS Prevention and Control by NGOs

NGO work on HIV/AIDS focuses on IEC and health promotion activities; work with young people and other vulnerable groups, particularly IDPs and refugees; testing; and the limited provision of testing and other commodities. Although the number of NGOs is increasing, relatively few address HIV/AIDS. There are only a few NGOs working with IDUs, which consistently report that the problem is much greater than presented in official figures. A few local NGOs are becoming advocates on issues related to MSM.

Table 44. NGO Sector in Serbia

Yugoslav Association Against AIDS (JAZAS)
- The oldest NGO on HIV/AIDS
- Involved in training of teachers and health professionals
- Organizes AIDS awareness campaigns
- Provides preventive activities for CSW

Youth of Yugoslav Association Against HIV/AIDS (Youth of JAZAS)
- The most active local NGO for HIV/AIDS in Serbia is Youth of JAZAS, established in 1994
- Has a large network of volunteers and educators with 10 branch offices in Serbia
- Trains educators on HIV/AIDS issues, dependence diseases, and leadership
- Organizes AIDS awareness campaigns
- Provides psychosocial support to PLWHA

ASTRA: Anti-Sex Trafficking Action: "Open Your Eyes"
- Belgrade-based NGO that works on human rights issues, particularly trafficking and women's rights

Yugoslav Medical Students International Committee
- Advocacy for better support and access to testing and treatment for PLWHA and peer-to-peer education

The Yugoslav Red Cross (YRC) with IFRC
- Conducts HIV/AIDS information campaigns
- Has developed HIV peer education

IOM
- Facilitates voluntary repatriation of trafficked women
- Carries out HIV testing for travelers if required by the country of destination
- Limited support is also provided through the AIDS SOS telephone hot line

---

The NGO sector is relatively new in Serbia and, therefore, would need initial support to be fully established and sustainable in order to complement gaps in social services. Bilateral donors support most NGOs, while some are also providing some of their own resources through fundraising activities.

Table 45. World Bank Support—Serbia

Projects that address HIV directly	Projects that could include HIV/AIDS action	Analytical work that addresses HIV or risk factors
	Trade and Transport Facilitation in Southeast Europe	
	Social Sector Adjustment	
	Social Sector Technical Assistance	
	Education Development	
	Health Investment Project	
	Essential Hospital Services	

Table 46. International Support—Serbia

UNAIDS TG	■ Help strengthening strategic response to HIV/AIDS and implementation of activities that lead towards accomplishment of goals set in Declaration of Commitment on HIV/AIDS of 2001
	■ Introduce a UN Learning Strategy on HIV/AIDS among UN Agencies
	■ With UNHCHR, review the legal framework and provide guidance on issues of social exclusion for PLWHA
	■ Participates in integrating HIV/AIDS in PRSP
	■ Manages coordination of HIV/AIDS stakeholders at republican levels
	■ Provides TA to Serbian GFATM-funded HIV/AIDS project
	■ Member of the Steering Committee of the DFID Initiative
	■ Provides assistance to the improvement of the HIV Surveillance System and capacity building of professionals
	■ Initiated establishment of a Monitoring and Evaluation Unit at the national/republican level
UNICEF	■ UNICEF RAR on especially vulnerable young people and Multiple Indicator Cluster Survey II 2000
	■ Technical partner for Serbia's approved GFATM grant
	■ Raising awareness and social mobilization on risks and prevention of HIV/AIDS/STIs
	■ Outreach with especially vulnerable young people at risk of HIV/AIDS/STIs
	■ Life skills-based education on HIV through peer education and other in and out of school interventions
	■ Establishing youth-friendly health services
	■ Strengthening capacities for voluntary confidential counseling and testing for HIV
	■ Provided 30,000 HIV test kits in 2000 and an additional 12,000 in 2001 to 14 institutions in Serbia and Montenegro
	Supported NGO peer education projects and drug prevention and HIV awareness activities
WHO	Technical partner for Serbia's approved GFATM grant
GFATM	Approved US$2,7 million over two years; grant agreement signed in April 2003. Grant is financing:
	■ Development of a national HIV strategy
	■ Education of health care staff
	■ HIV education at schools
	■ Social marketing of condoms
	■ PMTCT
	■ HIV prevention among high-risk groups
DFID	■ Finances the HIV Prevention Among Vulnerable Populations Initiative
	■ Advocacy
	■ Monitoring and evaluation
	■ Epidemiological and behavioral evidence on HIV risk behavior

Table 46. International Support—Serbia (*Continued*)

	▓ Provision of direct services to vulnerable populations, community organizing and advocacy
	▓ Develop capacity of up to eight HIV prevention demonstration projects across Serbia
	▓ The projects were launched in May 2004
CIDA	Under the Regional Strengthening of Essential Public Health Functions in the Balkans project, the Canadian Public Health Association has provided financial and technical assistance to:
	▓ Strengthen HIV/AIDS and STI surveillance systems in Serbia
	▓ Rapid Assessment of the surveillance system
	▓ Technical advice and training in surveillance methods and data analysis and interpretation
	▓ Support skills building in health promotion strategies and best practices related to voluntary counseling and testing, HIV prevention, and AIDS care and support
	▓ Mapping of care, support, and treatment process for PLWHA in Serbia
	▓ Establishment of the Serbian Public Health Association in 2003
USAID	▓ Supporting work on the surveillance system through CDC
EU CARDS	▓ Interethnic relations and civil society
	▓ Trade and private sector development
	▓ Infrastructure development
	▓ Reform of the judiciary
	▓ Integrated border management
	▓ Immigration and asylum
	▓ Fight against crime
EAR	▓ Improving medicine management practices in Serbia: €5.5 million
	▓ Support to Public Health development in Serbia: €2.5 million
	▓ Capacity building of MOH: €2 million
	▓ Establishment of and support to a National Blood Transfusion service in Serbia: €3 million
	▓ Rehabilitation of hospital and health center equipment: €5 million
	▓ Rationalization of the local pharmaceutical industry: €0.4 million
Others	▓ Additional support has been received from SIDA and the Netherlands and Finnish embassies

International Partner Organizations

Until 2003, there was limited donor funding for HIV/AIDS in Serbia, most of which was concentrated on preventive and education activities. However, the UNAIDS Theme Group, UNICEF, and the Canadian Public Health Association, financed by CIDA, had carried significant work in strategic, surveillance, and prevention areas; and local and international NGOs had undertaken some work with drug users. In 2003, Serbia obtained a grant from the Global Fund to Fight AIDS, TB and Malaria of $2.7 million. In addition, DFID is providing support for work with highly vulnerable groups, with a planned allocation of $2.6 million over two years. The HIV Prevention Among Populations Initiative (HPVPI) in Serbia and Montenegro started in 2004. Implementing partners for this Initiative are the Open Society Institute (New York), the Imperial College (London, UK), and the UNDP Belgrade Office.

The UNAIDS Theme Group in Serbia coordinates the national and regional efforts in strengthening capacity to fight against HIV/AIDS epidemic. The Work Plan for 2004 of the UNAIDS Theme Group had four components: (i) Support to national bodies dealing with HIV/AIDS; (ii) Improvement of the HIV surveillance system for Serbia and Montenegro, including development of the system for monitoring and evaluation of response to HIV/AIDS; (iii) National campaign; and (iv) Networking, coordination and national capacity building. Strong cooperation and coordination has been achieved among member agencies and local governmental and non-governmental partners. UNAIDS Geneva allocated funds from the Program Accelerating Fund (PAF) for some programmatic activities of the UNTG in 2004-2005. However, despite the fact that the workload has significantly increased for the UN Theme Group in recent years, its basic operations have been jeopardized by lack of funding. It is urgent that a solution to this situation is found, primarily with the support of UN agencies working in Serbia.

The objective of the Bank-supported Health Project is to build a sustainable, performance-oriented health care system. In addition, the goal is to support the planning and initial implementation of the Government's strategy to improve the efficiency of health-care delivery while maintaining quality. It also aims at ensuring access to affordable and effective care through increased health insurance coverage. The Project does not include a Public Health Component, nor HIV/AIDS activities.

CHAPTER 10

Profile: Montenegro

Table 47. Epidemiology—Montenegro

Population	650,000
Registered HIV cases	65
Registered AIDS cases IPH 2004	35
HIV/AIDS Prevalence	<0.1
New HIV Cases IPH 2004	NA
Modes of Transmission IHP 2004	▓ Heterosexual 50% ▓ Homosexual 25%
Registered STIs cases IHP 2004	▓ Syphilis: 19 cases in 1990–2002 ▓ Gonorrhea: 181 cases (1992–2002)
TB notification rate	NA
Vulnerable Groups UNICEF RAR 2002	Youth ▓ 20% of population between 15–24 IDU ▓ Mean age 19 ▓ 67% IDUs have 2–5 sex partners per year MSM ▓ NA Mobile population ▓ 14% infections among sailors ▓ 6% sailors tested HIV positive ▓ Sailors have multiple sex partners ▓ 14% infections among tourist workers ▓ Over 200,000 tourists every season ▓ High seasonal migration for employment abroad ▓ High influx of refugees

Epidemiological Overview: HIV/AIDS and STIS

HIV/AIDS

The first HIV infection in Montenegro was reported in 1989. Since then through December 2004, 55 HIV infections have been recorded. Of these, 35 have developed AIDS; of them, 24 have died. Among the AIDS cases, the male to female ratio is 3:1 and 90 percent are in the 25–49 age group. HIV prevalence is thought to be at least 10 times higher than the reported number, which would be between 500 and 800 cases. Approximately 75 percent of reported cases are transmitted sexually; of this, heterosexual transmission accounts for 50 percent, and homo/bisexual for 25 percent. About 14 percent of all cases occurred among tourist workers and another 14 percent among sailors. Geographically, one-third of all cases are from Podgorica and almost one-half from coastal municipalities.

Sexually-transmitted Infections

There were 19 registered cases of syphilis in the last 12 years, and there have been long periods with no cases recorded. These numbers seem impossibly low as a realistic measure within this population and may point to extremely incomplete notification or case definition. The official notifications of syphilis in Montenegro from 1990–2002 are shown in Table 48.

Since 1990, 181 cases of gonorrhea have been reported. In 1990, the incidence rate was 1.9 per 100,000 population. In the last five years, there were 12 cases per year on average, whereas during the 1990–1994 period, there were 16 cases per year on average. Incidence has been low and a slight decrease in the current overall trend is noticeable. The most affected group was men aged 20–39, who made up over 75 percent of the total number of cases. About 15 percent of all cases were men and women below the age of 20 (4 women and 22 men). Only 10 cases among all registered cases were women and the overall ratio of men to women was 17:1. Again, these numbers seem impossibly low as a realistic measure within this population and points to extremely incomplete notification. The official notifications of gonorrhea in Montenegro from 1990–2002 are shown in Table 49. No data are available on chlamydia.

Table 48. Notified Syphilis Cases in Montenegro, 1990–2002

| Year | No. of Notified cases | | |
| | Total | Gender | |
		Men	Women
1990	0	0	0
1991	0	0	0
1992	2	1	1
1993	2	1	1
1994	2	2	0
1995	2	2	0
1996	2	2	0
1997	2	2	0
1998	0	0	0
1999	0	0	0
2000	0	0	0
2001	3	2	1
2002	4	3	1
Total	19	15	4

Source: IPH 2003.

Vulnerability to HIV/AIDS: Contextual Factors

In 2003, Montenegro had a population of approximately 650,000 people, out of which about 5 percent were internally displaced, refugees, and Roma. In April 1992, the Federal Republic of Yugoslavia (FRY) was formed as the self-proclaimed successor to the Socialist Federal Republic of Yugoslavia. In February 2003, the FRY Parliament adopted a new constitutional charter establishing the Federal Union of Serbia and Montenegro, comprising the Republic of Serbia and the Republic of Montenegro. Under the provisions of the new constitutional charter, Serbia and Montenegro (SaM) have some joint institutions, including the Presidency, Parliament, and a Council of Ministers, but operate separate economic, fiscal, monetary, and customs policies.

Table 49. Notified Cases of Gonorrhea in Montenegro 1990–2002

Year	Total	Men	Women
	No. of Notified cases		
		Gender	
1990	20	20	0
1991	17	17	0
1992	16	14	2
1993	10	10	0
1994	19	19	0
1995	21	18	3
1996	14	12	2
1997	6	6	0
1998	10	10	0
1999	14	14	0
2000	14	11	3
2001	8	8	0
2002	12	12	0
Total	181	171	10

Source: IPH 2003.

Economy

About 6 percent of the population, and 20 percent of the workforce, are public service employees, including health care employees—one of the highest levels in Europe. Montenegro's economy is oriented toward tourism, trade, shipbuilding, naval transportation, and agriculture, as well as small- and medium-sized enterprise (Wong 2002b). Every season, there are approximately 200,000 visitors to Montenegro, who are served by tourist workers primarily from the coastal cities but also from other parts of Montenegro and from Serbia (Rhodes and others 2003). Although providing economic opportunities, the transport and tourism sectors also entail increases in mobility, possible regroupings of family units, and exposure to new sexual networks, which may have significant ramifications for HIV transmission.

Poverty

Recent poverty surveys point to the vulnerability of Montenegrin youth. Using a poverty threshold level in an average region of Montenegro at € 3.50 a day shows that 9.4 percent of the population falls below the poverty line. However, over 25 percent of the population has a consumption that is only precariously above the poverty line; increasing the poverty line by 10 percent raises poverty at both the household and individual levels by approximately one-third, indicating that even small economic shocks can have potentially large effects on poverty. A Poverty Assessment was carried out in 2003 (World Bank 2003e, 2003h).

The level of unemployment is high. The unemployed in Montenegro are predominantly in their late twenties. In a sample surveyed in 2001, four-fifths of the unemployed were people with secondary education. According to the data of the Employment Office, only 3 percent of registered unemployed people received benefits. Close to 33 percent of the employed are working without an employment contract, meaning that around 30 percent most likely do not have access to health services.

A pattern of gender discrimination is present in the Montenegrin economy. Women are more often unemployed or economically inactive than men. In addition, they are more often involved in informal activities, and comparatively less involved in multiple and formal types of employment, which are relatively well-paid (Government of the Republic of Montenegro 2002).

Mobility

Montenegro has been experiencing a strong level of mobility. High numbers of people from other countries enter Montenegro on a regular basis. For example, the tourism industry brings in a high number of tourists, which increases the risk to youth and tourist workers. In addition, Montenegro is the place of residence of many thousands of refugees and IDPs, who often live in poor conditions and represents vulnerable groups for STIs and HIV/AIDS. To date, no systematic strategies have been developed for working with these populations and the experience of other countries indicates they are all vulnerable groups. For their part, Montenegrins travel extensively for economic reasons, often to and from countries where there is a higher prevalence of HIV/AIDS. High migrations present one of the major risks for HIV infection for Montenegro. Increasingly higher economic

Table 50. Vulnerability Factors—Montenegro

GNI per Capita CIDA. 2002	US$1,400 (Serbia and Montenegro)
Unemployment World Bank. 2003	▨ Majority of unemployed in their late 20s ▨ More women unemployed than men ▨ 80% unemployed with secondary education
Poverty Government. 2002 **Mobility**	▨ 9.4% ▨ 14% HIV infections among sailors ▨ 14% infections among tourist workers ▨ 200,000 tourists per season
Trafficking	▨ No quantitative data available on trafficking victims ▨ Major route to Western Europe for trafficked victims ▨ No laws against trafficking

migration was reported during the last decade. Naval transportation is also a major industry for Montenegro, adding to the high level of economic migration. The high influx of refugees and strong number of economic migration result in an increased average age of the population. This, combined with the epidemiological shift in predominance from communicable to non-communicable diseases, is creating higher demands and costs for health services.

Vulnerable Groups

Although HIV prevalence is low, Montenegro has identifiable factors that put the population at risk. A high level of mobility of both Montenegrins out of the territory and other nationalities into Montenegro is a major issue that can affect multiple vulnerable groups at risk.

Youth. One fifth of the population in Montenegro is between 15 and 24 years of age. Conflict, poverty, and high unemployment, combined with deteriorating economic conditions, and a decline in public service provision and infrastructure, are likely to contribute to increased risk practices among young people. Programs that promote young people's health have been inconsistently implemented. For example, in 2001, the Montenegrin Government adopted the Action Plan for Drug Abuse Prevention with Children and Young Adults in Montenegro, which identified drug addiction as the top priority for young people's health. Yet, since the formal adoption of the program, little has been done in terms of actual implementation. Health services for young people in the areas of reproductive and mental health are inaccessible and insufficient; furthermore, there is a lack of interest within the community to address these issues. In addition, there are insufficient services that address the issues of drugs and HIV/AIDS. Drug and HIV/AIDS prevention programs exist in primary schools, but not in high schools or by the faculties.

Sailors and Tourist Industry Workers. As mentioned previously, 14 percent of recorded HIV infections in Montenegro have occurred among tourist workers and 14 percent among sailors. Every season, there are approximately 200,000 visitors to Montenegro served by tourist workers primarily from the coastal cities but also from other parts of Montenegro and from Serbia. Although the transport and tourism sectors provide economic opportunities, they also entail an increase in mobility, possible regroupings of family units, and exposure to new sexual networks, which may have significant ramifications for HIV transmission.

Sailors are at high risk for infection due to their lifestyle. The UNICEF RAR stated that while sailors are on travel duty, they visit brothels and have multiple sexual partners, as well as engage in alcohol and drug use. Almost every fourth sailor reported experience with drugs and every third had sex under the effects of drugs. Every sixth sailor reported using a condom regularly. Despite the high-risk behavior, only 6 percent of sailors have been tested for HIV. While limited health protection for sailors exists at home, it is not specifically adapted to their needs. There are no advisory services for sailors from Montenegro that offer all forms of health protection. On board ship, they turn to self-medication. Sailors reported that they were more afraid of malaria than AIDS. The STI and HIV/AIDS information that they received in their regular studies was inadequate. Before boarding ship, sailors would have liked more information on STIs and HIV/AIDS. There was a sense that the majority of sailors use alcohol and drugs because of boredom (Wong 2002b).

Additionally, the DFID HIV Prevention Among Vulnerable Populations Initiative in Serbia and Montenegro (Rhodes and others 2003) suggests that there is a heightened risk of the Montenegrin population mixing with those abroad due to the recent closure of two naval transport companies in Montenegro. This has resulted in thousands of workers losing their jobs and having to find new work abroad, in a number of companies all over the world. There is a concern that the risks of HIV transmission for sailors will intensify because of the decline in the naval transport industry over the past decade. DFID also found that free condoms are not readily available to sailors and tourist industry workers. Free condoms tend to be available only in the two weeks surrounding World AIDS Day. Finally, DFID states that there is a prevailing conservative culture of shame in Montenegro related to most aspects of sex life.

Sex Workers and Trafficking. Montenegro is one of the main routes for women being trafficked to Western Europe, due to loosely controlled borders and the weaknesses of the authorities to effectively combat international organized crime. Although Montenegro is predominantly an area of transition, in recent years, it has also become a destination for trafficked women. However, there is little information available regarding the scale and dimension of trafficking in human beings in Montenegro. There are neither clear laws against trafficking nor any clear understanding of the issue by the authorities. Moreover, there is alleged complicity on the part of the police and judiciary, especially at the local level. The sex industry in Montenegro is largely organized around bars, clubs, and motels in the capital and coastal cities.

MSM. There is little information on men who have sex with men. Similar to other countries in the region, the gay and bisexual community is largely underground and not politically mobilized.

Drug Users. The incidence of IDU in Montenegro is reported to be low, and sharing injection equipment is uncommon according to UNICEF's RAR. The DFID HIV Prevention Among Vulnerable Populations Initiative in Montenegro confirmed that the spread of heroin in Montenegro was more recent than had been the case in Serbia. The diffusion of drug use was associated with the recent growth in tourism. While acknowledging an increased diffusion of drug use (including heroin), interviewees responded that injecting drug use was relatively less common in Montenegro than in Serbia. They described injecting drug use among Montenegrin drug users as "unpopular," indicating that they were more accustomed to snorting or smoking heroin or using non-injectable drugs such as pills, cannabis, hashish, or cocaine (Rhodes and ohters 2003).

Among young people who use drugs but do not inject, the UNICEF RAR found that the initial use of drugs was not due to peer pressure but due to solidarity within the group and the curiosity to experience something new. Young people used drugs to help overcome unpleasant realities. The participants did not feel that using cannabis would damage their health or lead to the use of harder drugs. Cannabis is easily accessible. It is sold on the streets, in cafes, and around schools. Cannabis is often consumed in public places, although as drug use becomes more severe (for example, using heroin), the most common place for using drugs is the home. It usually takes about two years to go from using cannabis to heroin. Participants in this study reported that they could recognize a safe sexual partner by his/her "tidy" looks. Most did not use condoms with their steady partner. If a condom was used, it was usually for the purpose of contraception rather than for protection against STIs. Condoms were not openly discussed among youth and were not used often because of shame, although they can be purchased at pharmacies (Wong 2002b).

In 1999, the Institute of Public Health, the Ministry of Education and Science and UNICEF undertook a survey among schoolchildren between the ages of 11 and 18. More than 70 percent of the surveyed students stated that drugs were used in school, mostly marijuana (18 percent) and pills (12 percent), while the use of other drugs was insignificant. Drugs were more present in high schools than in primary schools. About 73 percent reported obtaining drugs with pocket money, 23 percent through theft, and 14 percent through prostitution. About 67 percent of IDUs reported sharing drug-using equipment and 89 percent of IDUs had sex under the influence of drugs, but only 13 percent reported always using condoms. Over half (56 percent) of the respondents reported having been tested for HIV. Even among youth not using drugs, 40 percent had multiple partners in the past year and only half always used condoms.

Roma. According to official estimates (2003 census), there are about 12,000 Roma in Montenegro, most living in two separate camps. Roma have very poor access to health service; concurrently, demand for health services by Roma appears to be very low. Almost 33 percent of Roma women have never visited a general practice doctor and more than 90 percent have never visited a gynecologist, even though 80 percent of married women have more than four children.

HIV/AIDS Awareness and Knowledge

Research performed by IPH indicates that basic knowledge about HIV and STIs in Montenegro among school-age children is very low. Less knowledge and awareness of HIV/AIDS is observed in rural areas. Overall, HIV/AIDS awareness among health professionals appears to be low, and no protection or prevention strategies for health workers are available at heath facilities.

Health Care in Montenegro

Montenegro has a well-established public health and clinical care infrastructure. Health care services are provided through a large network of government-owned facilities, comprising 21 primary care health centers; 7 general hospitals and 5 health stations at the secondary level; and the Clinical Center Podgorica as well as three special hospitals and the Institute for Medical Rehabilitation at the tertiary level. Outpatient health protection and public health services are provided by the Health Institute of Montenegro. Public facilities do not have independent budgets, and expenditures for an unsustainably generous benefits package are reimbursed by the HIF. Hence, there are no incentives for efficient use of the system. In addition to the public system, there are about 117 private health institutions and

Table 51. UNICEF's Rapid Assessment and Response in Montenegro 2002

	Drug users	IDU	Youth (%)	Sailors
Mean age in years	20	19	18	20
Mean age at first drug use	16	17	—	18
Had sexual intercourse (%)	92	89	35	80
Thought they were at risk of HIV or other STIs (%)	45	56	39	50
Tested for HIV (%)	8.5	56	1.1	6
Used in the past month (%)				
Alcohol	75	56	—	93
Cannabis	66	78	—	93
Diazepam	21	33	—	
Analgesics	8.5	—	—	
Heroin	—	44	—	
Ecstasy	—	33	—	
Cocaine	—	—	14	
Shared drug-injecting equipment (%)	—	67	—	No IDUs
Used 2 or more drugs at the same time (%)	60	100	—	43
Had sex under the influence of drugs (%)	66	89	—	36
Mean age at first sexual intercourse	16	15	16	17
Had 1 sexual partner in the past year (%)	21	—	46	48
Had between 2 and 5 sexual partners in the past year (%)	65	67	40	43
Always used condoms during sex (%)	26	12.5	51	37
Sometimes or never used condoms during sex (%)	72	78	51	63
Had sex in return for money, drugs (%)	14	33.	7	10
Reasons for not always using condoms during sex	—Do not like sex with condoms —Trust in partners —Difficult to use	—Condoms are expensive to purchase —Do not like sex with condoms —Condoms are not easily available —STI	—Trust in partners —Do not like sex with condoms —Embarrassed to ask partners to use condoms	—Do not like sex with condoms —Trust in partners
Sources of information about HIV or other STIs	—Friends or peers —Media —Family	counseling services —Family —Media	—Media —Friends or peers —Family	—Media —Friends or peers —Family

Source: Wong 2002b.

Table 52. Knowledge, Attitudes, and Practices—Montenegro

Youth UNICEF RAR	▨ Very low basic knowledge about HIV/AIDS among school-age children ▨ 56% of students refer multiple sex partners ▨ 50% of them refer always using condoms
IDU UNICEF RAR	▨ Condoms considered contraception ▨ 12,5% who have 2–5 sex partners per year refer always using condoms ▨ Others not using condoms because of high cost
Health staff	▨ HIV/AIDS awareness among health professionals appears to be low ▨ No protection or prevention strategies for health workers at heath facilities

ambulances (but no private pharmacies) that offer their services in Montenegro. Payments for these services are out of pocket or covered from private health insurance schemes.

The major constraints facing Montenegro's health system include (World Bank 2004):

▨ Public and private health expenditure is high, and the current public health financing and delivery system is not financially sustainable because of insufficient revenue (contribution waivers, difficulty collecting from the informal sector, lack of budget transfers for the uninsured, including refugees and IDPs) and high expenditure (through failure to adjust the benefits package and capacity to reduced economic circumstances).

▨ Pharmaceutical expenditure is at almost 30 percent of HIF expenditure, plus widespread out-of-pocket payment. Drug prices are significantly above international reference prices.

▨ Capacity for policy development, planning, forecasting, managing, and monitoring the system is weak and fragmented, and information systems and data for these functions are deficient.

▨ Primary health care (PHC) is not playing a sufficient role in prevention or diagnosis and treatment, and staff is not optimally distributed, creating access problems in some places despite PHC employing a large share of health sector staff. Organization of PHC is fragmented and overlaps with hospital care. Reform of PHC based on a family-medicine model has been considered as an option to address some of these problems, but has become controversial.

▨ Health sector staff is poorly paid, motivated, and managed; inadequately trained; and often work to low standards. Unregulated private practice, financed by out-of-pocket payments, and informal payments in the public sector have emerged spontaneously in response to these problems, to the detriment of access to care. There is no framework for the HIF to contract with the private sector or for private supplementary insurance, and there has been no privatization of public services.

■ Health and social care services for the growing proportion of the elderly and for those with chronic mental illness and disabilities are limited. The interface with the responsibilities of the Ministry of Social Affairs and Labor needs to be clarified.

■ The network of public hospitals and the Republic Institute of Public Health are "run-down" and inefficient. Standards need to be defined and improved.

Funding of Health Services

With over 23 percent of GDP spent on social protection and health ($150 per capita), Montenegro has one of the highest expenditures for these sectors in the region (World Bank 2002e). At the same time, public investments are low and many public services are either of poor quality or inefficient. Public spending in the health sector alone is around 10 percent of GDP, which is also one of the highest in the region, compared to countries with similar income. As Montenegro does not have an excess number of medical staff or health facilities as measured by EU standards, the high level of health expenditures suggests significant inefficiencies in the sector.

Public health care financing was mainly from the HIF (95 percent came from earmarked contributions). The remainder comprised MOH spending and spending of the then Yugoslav National Army in Montenegro. Total national health spending in 2001 amounted to an estimated $65 million, or about $92 per capita. The Government of Montenegro contributed 8 percent of its total budget to health care and health care systems in 2001. There are no official figures on private health expenditures, including out-of-pocket health payments. A UNDP survey in 2000 and 2001 estimated that 25 percent of the total health expenditure (approximately 3 percent of GDP), was for private spending. Of this amount, approximately one-fourth was for official co-payments, and three-fourths was for private services and drugs.

Contributions to the Health Insurance Fund are raised through a payroll tax on salaries and wages. The Health Insurance Fund provides universal coverage of the population. However, links between contributions and benefits are weak, and an inadequate incentive structure for efficient service provision has led to a funding gap between HIF revenues and expenditures, resulting in debts. As a consequence, the HIF has significant arrears.

Funding for HIV/AIDS

There is no specific allocation of funds for HIV/AIDS prevention and testing services in the budgets of the MOH and HIF so far. The costs of testing HIV (about $300,000 in 2001) and ARV treatments are covered in the budget allocation for communicable diseases. Funding of HIV/AIDS-related activities has competed with other priorities, particularly because the total number of HIV and AIDS cases up to now has been relatively small. The estimated Government and donor funding for HIV/AIDS from 2001 to 2006 is shown below.

Total available resources for HIV/AIDS services in Montenegro in 2001 amounted to approximately $477,100. This contrasts sharply with the estimated funding requirements of around $780,000 to provide basic comprehensive services to target HIV/AIDS for that year. The application to the GFATM was not approved in 2003 and 2004, which leaves Montenegro with a resource gap of around 68 percent of Government-estimated total

Table 53. Estimated Resource Needs and Funding Gaps for HIV/AIDS Treatment, Montenegro

	2001	2004	2005	2006
Government allocation (1)	313,500	350,000	400,000	600,000
Donor allocation (1)	183,000	45,000		
Total funding for HIV/AIDS (1)	496,500	395,000	400,000	600,000
Resource Needs (2)	1,255,484	1,274,983	1,429,816	1,228,200
Funding Gap	758,984	879,983	1,029,816	628,200

Source: (1) GFATM application, (2) WB/UNAIDS estimates. Study estimates used the total population of 709,313 as denominator.

requirements in 2004, 72 percent in 2005 and half of the funds required for activities in 2006, or a total of US$2.5 million. This gap is expected to widen over the next couple of years as funding needs will increase with the rise of the epidemic, and sustaining present Government funding appears uncertain, particularly in light of recent expenditure cuts.

Thus, in order to prevent the spread of the disease in the near future, there is great urgency for the Government to initiate further fundraising activities, mobilize other resources, and work at the re-allocation of public funds to ensure the provision of adequate HIV/AIDS preventive and curative services. Table 53 summarizes the resources available in 2001, as well as the estimated needs for HIV/AIDS funding for the next three years.

Government and Civil Society Action on HIV/AIDS

Strategic, Policy, and Regulatory Framework

In 2001, Montenegro established the Republican AIDS Commission (RAC), which seeks to address HIV/AIDS in a multisectoral fashion, and works closely with the UNTG on HIV/AIDS for Serbia and Montenegro. In 2002, the Commission began a strategic planning process on HIV/AIDS (UNAIDS 2003d). The RCA includes representatives from the Ministries of Health, Education, Justice, Social Welfare, Tourism, and Interior; representatives of the Montenegrin Institute of Public Health, Department of Communicable Diseases of the Montenegrin Clinical Centre/Primary Care Centre; and members of Montenegrin NGOs. The Government has also established Country Coordination Mechanism, consisting of RCA members and UNDP, UNICEF, WHO and UNAIDS TG representatives. The CCM purpose is to prepare a grant proposal to submit to the GFATM, and monitor its implementation.

In 2003 and 2004, the CCM submitted detailed grant proposals to the GFATM, which have not been approved. Although there are few broad-based HIV/AIDS prevention activities in Montenegro, collaboration between UN agencies and the MOH is good. Montenegrin health officials have recently acknowledged that a significant gap exists in provision of HIV/AIDS service and treatment, and have begun to take measures to improve the situation (IOM and UNICEF 2002). Following his participation in the Dublin meeting in March

2004, the Minister of Health has stated his intention of completing an HIV/AIDS strategy for Government and Parliament approval by the end of 2004.

Currently, there is no specific legal framework to protect the rights of PLWHA in Montenegro. However, UNHCHR and the UN Theme Group on HIV/AIDS are examining legal frameworks to incorporate a human rights approach (IOM and UNICEF 2002). The Technical Commission on Substance Abuse, formed in 2001, is an inter-ministerial working group of professionals. Its work focuses on research and prevention of substance abuse in Montenegro.

The Montenegro Institute of Public Health is planning to address the lack of awareness regarding HIV/AIDS among health professionals. One initiative highlights closer cooperation and an exchange program with the HIV/AIDS Center at the Institute for Infectious and Tropical Diseases Clinical University Center in Belgrade. Other initiatives planned by the IPH would require professionals to accept and follow universal precautions (which in turn require funding for the provision of appropriate supplies). Presently, the IPH runs a program to prevent substance abuse in all the elementary schools in Podgorica, and monitors the health status of IDPs in camps and collective centers.

HIV/AIDS and STIs Surveillance

Montenegro's Institute of Public Health, including its laboratory and epidemiological divisions, has a national statutory responsibility for prevention and surveillance of infectious

---

Table 54. Government Intervention and Institutional Arrangements—Montenegro

Intersectoral coordination	▨ The Republican AIDS Commission (RAC) includes representatives from the Government, IPH and NGOs
	▨ The Commission on Substance Abuse is an inter-ministerial working group established in 2001
National HIV/AIDS Strategy and Legislation	▨ An Action Plan for Drug Abuse Prevention with Children and Young Adults was developed in 2001 but has not been implemented
	▨ The GFATM application has been rejected twice
	▨ Following participation in the Dublin meeting in March 2004, the Minister of Health has stated the intention of completing and HIV/AIDS strategy for approval by the end of 2004
	▨ Resource gap of $2.5 million
	▨ No specific legal framework to protect the rights of PLWHA
	▨ Intervention projects with high risk groups such as migrants, CSW and IDU have not been yet been developed in the public sector
Government institution responsible for HIV/AIDS	▨ The Republican AIDS Commission seeks to address HIV/AIDS in a multisectoral fashion and works closely with the UNAIDS-TG
	▨ The Republican Institute of Public Health (IPH) is responsible for prevention and surveillance of HIV/AIDS and STIs

and chronic diseases, including HIV/AIDS and STIs. Although there are no other IPHs in Montenegro, there are 21 district Primary Health Centers (PHCs) with a statutory responsibility for reporting 70 notifiable infectious diseases, including HIV/AIDS, gonorrhea, syphilis, chlamydia, Hepatitis A and Hepatitis B. The Montenegrin IPH regularly produces HIV surveillance reports.

Reporting infectious diseases is regulated by the acts set out in the Official Gazette of FRY 27/97. It stipulates that reporting STIs is based on clinical or laboratory diagnosis and is done by the diagnosing physician, who fills out a pre-printed form and sends it to the IPH within 24 hours of diagnosis. The pre-printed form does not ask for the risk group, only for occupation. However, it is generally believed that STI reporting is poor, especially by physicians in the private sector where most STIs are treated, due to the fear of loss of confidentiality and subsequent stigma. Many public health laboratory-confirmed STI cases are not reported either. Also, there have been instances of reporting delays from district epidemiological units to Montenegro IPH.

HIV testing is available in eight general hospitals as well as at the IPH in Podgorica. HIV testing is free of cost with a referral letter from a physician; otherwise it costs about €7.50. IOM offers testing for people who are emigrating overseas and a HIV test is a prerequisite for travel to several countries. Anonymous HIV testing is illegal and unavailable, but advocacy for introducing it has been initiated. Pre- and post-test counseling is limited (Wong 2002b). Patients with active TB or STIs are not routinely tested for HIV. Finally, it is compulsory for all donated blood to be screened.

Since 2001, the Montenegro IPH has developed the capacity to perform HIV Western Blot confirmatory testing (Wong 2002b). All positive HIV cases are reported by name with risk information. Citizenship information is currently collected from foreigners. Pregnancy status is not requested in the standard form. However, the number of positive HIV test reports captures only those who came forward for testing, were diagnosed with HIV infection, and were then reported. Only a small number of individuals pursue voluntary HIV testing because of the stigma and confidentiality concerns. At least 67 percent of newly reported HIV cases present at the AIDS level, raising concerns that individuals wait until the advanced stages of HIV/AIDS before coming forward for testing.

For confidentiality reasons, many residents go to Serbia to get tested for HIV. In Serbia, HIV testing (including confirmatory testing) is available in both the private and public system. If HIV testing is performed in the public system in Serbia, positive results will be reported to Montenegro. However, if HIV testing is done in the private laboratory system in Serbia, positive cases are not necessarily reported in Montenegro.

Laboratory tests for STI diagnosis are available but it is not clear to what extent. Individuals suspected of having an STI may be referred to a specialist by their doctor. Diagnosis will then be by laboratory testing, where available. Patients will also be asked to visit an epidemiologist (contact tracer) for the purpose of epidemiological analysis and partner notification. Most of the referred patients do meet with the epidemiologist and subsequent testing of partners is carried out in 40–50 percent of the cases. Clinical management of STIs is distributed through clinics and primary care structures throughout the territory. It is highly probable that management of STI diagnosis and treatment is largely syndromic. The extent to which rational protocols are used to guide management is uncertain.

Table 55. Government Intervention and Institutional Arrangements—Montenegro

Testing	▓ Anonymous HIV testing was illegal and unavailable in 2003
	▓ No allocation of funding for testing in MOH and HIF
	▓ HIV testing is available in 8 general hospitals and IPH in Podgorica
	▓ HIV testing is free of cost with a referral letter from a physician, otherwise costs about €7.5
	▓ IOM offers testing for people who are emigrating
	▓ Pre- and posttest counseling is limited
	▓ Patients with active TB or STIs are not routinely tested for HIV
	▓ HIV testing done in a private laboratory in Serbia is not reported
Surveillance	▓ Serious weaknesses of surveillance system
	▓ Atmosphere of stigma and discrimination around HIV/AIDS prevents individuals from admitting certain risk behavior
HIV/AIDS Notification	▓ 21 District Primary Health Centers are responsible for reporting HIV/AIDS cases to IPH
	▓ Many public health laboratory-confirmed STI cases are not reported
Blood Safety	▓ 4 HIV cases have been found, 2 from Podgorica
	▓ All donated blood is compulsory screened using quick test methods
	▓ Western Blot available at the IPH in Podgorica
Prevention	▓ No special allocation of funding for HIV/AIDS prevention in MOH and HIF
	▓ IPH runs a program to prevent substance abuse in elementary schools in Podgorica
	▓ IPH monitors the health status of IDPs in camps and collective centers
Treatment	▓ Patients referred to the HIV/AIDS Center at the Institute for Infectious and Tropical Diseases Clinical University Center in Belgrade
	▓ The Government health care system finances treatment for opportunistic infections for HIV+ patients

HIV/AIDS, STIs, and Drug Prevention and Control Use in the Public System

Intervention projects with high-risk groups such as migrants, CSW, and IDU have not yet been developed in the public sector. Additionally, there are no protection or prevention strategies for health workers in health facilities. Hospitals and clinics do not have proper protective equipment to reduce the risk of exposure, particularly for those in the transfusion centers, where the possibility of contact with contaminated blood is high. Access to basic supplies such as gloves and masks is limited and no PEP kits are available. Further, clinical waste disposal also remains a problem despite recent initiatives to resolve this problem.

Presently, the Ministry of Education and Science runs a program to prevent substance abuse in all elementary schools in Podgorica, and monitors the health status of IDPs in camps and collective centers (IOM and UNICEF 2002). The Program for Prevention of

Drug Addiction has been implemented throughout Montenegro since 2002. This program focuses on prevention of drug addiction and sexually-transmitted infections and is expected to reach 34,000 students in 105 elementary schools. Sexual health and STI occurrence is unknown among migrant populations, commercial sex workers, injecting drug users, and other groups at risk of HIV infection. However, there are likely to be significant problems.

HIV/AIDS and STIs Treatment

Presently, only STIs and symptomatic opportunistic infections are treated in Montenegro, at local public and private clinics and hospitals. The Podgorica Hospital of Infectious Diseases does not have a department for HIV/AIDS and no facilities to treat patients with HIV/AIDS; nor does it have facilities for CD4 count or PCR. Therefore, patients are referred to the HIV/AIDS Center at the Institute for Infectious and Tropical Diseases Clinical University Center in Belgrade. Unavailability of treatment in Montenegro creates an additional burden for Montenegrin PLWHA. For example, to receive reimbursement from the Health Insurance Fund, patients must obtain a prescription from a Montenegrin physician, purchase the drugs in Belgrade, and then request reimbursement from the Montenegrin HIF.

Currently, within the public health system, no network of specialized venereal or dermato-venereal diseases clinics operate within the territory. Diagnosis and treatment is carried out by primary care services and by specialists at urology centers for men and gynecology centers for women. The specialized dermatology and venereal diseases service now deals mostly with skin diseases. Most STI patients are treated in a few private clinics because they guarantee confidentiality. Availability of drugs for STI treatment is uncertain.

HIV/AIDS Prevention and Control by NGOs

Over the past several years, the number of NGOs in Podgorica has increased significantly, although very few provide support services targeted at young people (Wong 2002b). There are a few NGOs working on prevention of HIV/AIDS and drug use in Montenegro. Further strengthening of NGOs as well as fundraising activities is urgently required to improve services in this area. A summary of the main NGO activities is listed below.

Table 56. NGO Sector in Montenegro

- CAZAS is leading the work in the sector with funding from UNICEF and USAID, mainly for IEC activities and awareness campaigns. Carries out peer group education in high schools.
- The Montenegrin Red Cross has programs for prevention of drugs addition, HIV/AIDS and reproductive health.
- IPPF supports the NGO Juventus
- Overall funding for NGO activities in 200 amounted to $5,400

Table 57. World Bank Support—Montenegro

Projects that address HIV directly	Projects that could include HIV/AIDS action	Analytical work that addresses HIV or risk factors
	Montenegro Health System Improvement	

International Partner Organizations

Total donor commitments for 2004 for HIV/AIDS were expected to be around $45,000, or 3.5 percent of the total funding needed for HIV/AIDS. Donor support in 2001 amounted to approximately $158,000, of which $120,000 came from UNICEF for IEC activities and

Table 58. International Support—Montenegro

UNTG	▓ Operational in 2000
Serbia and Montenegro	▓ Advocates for Government commitment and coordinated response towards HIV/AIDS and establishment of the RCA
	▓ Assist development of a Republican AIDS Strategy
	▓ Assist the development of a grant proposal for submission to GFATM
	▓ Assist improvement of HIV Surveillance System and development of System for Monitoring and evaluation of response on HIV/AIDS, and introduction of Country Response Information System (CRIS)
UNICEF	▓ In co-operation with CPHA and Health Canada, conducted the Rapid Assessment of youth and sailors awareness
CIDA	▓ The Canadian Public Health Association (CPHA) has provided technical assistance for the elaboration of the Global Fund proposal on HIV prevention, and for a review of laboratory management and operations
	▓ Rapid assessment of a Montenegro HIV/AIDS and STI surveillance system, which provides the most exhaustive, up-to date surveillance information
DFID	▓ Finances the HIV Prevention Among Populations Initiative (HPVPI)
$2.6 million for Serbia and Montenegro	▓ Implementing partners are Open Society Institute (New York) and Imperial College (London, UK)
	▓ The Initiative will fund and develop capacity of up to four HIV prevention demonstration projects across Serbia and Montenegro.
	▓ Projects will provide direct services to vulnerable populations, community organization, and advocacy
	▓ The epidemiological and behavioral evidence base of HIV risk behavior, and the intervention coverage among vulnerable populations from a few sites will be included.

technical assistance for the Rapid Assessment. UNICEF's funding was reduced to $20,000 in 2002. The limited donor funding for HIV/AIDS in Montenegro concentrated mostly on awareness and education activities, mainly through local and international NGOs on the ground. Multi-sectoral partnerships on HIV/AIDS began to develop in Montenegro in 2000.

The World Bank is financing the Montenegro Health System Improvement, which focuses on stabilizing health financing and improving primary health care. However, the Project does not include improvements in public health not HIV/AIDS activities.

CHAPTER 11

Profile: Kosovo

Table 59. Epidemiology—Kosovo	
Population	2.4 million
NIS 2003	
Registered HIV/AIDS cases	61
NIPH 2004	
HIV/AIDS Prevalence	<0.1
UNAIDS 2003	
New HIV Cases	1999— 4
NIPH 2004	2000—6
	2001—12
	2002—5
	2003—7
	2004—7
Modes of Transmission	Heterosexual transmission
Registered STIs cases	▓ All STI—2,093 (1990–2004)
NIPH 2004	▓ Gonorrhea—6 (2004)
	▓ Chlamydia—405 (2004)
	▓ Syphilis—6 (2001–2002)
TB notification rate	▓ Hepatitis B—1009 (2001–2004)
NIPH 2004	▓ 48 per 100,000

(continued)

Table 59. Epidemiology—Kosovo (*Continued*)

Vulnerable Groups	Youth
IOM, UNICEF, UNDP 2003–2004	▓ 57% of population under 25
	▓ Enrolment in secondary education 75%
	▓ Injecting drugs increasing among youth
	Injecting Drug Users
	▓ Key transit route of heroin into Europe
	▓ Over 5,000 heroin users
	▓ Sharing of needles high
	▓ All of 20 hospitalized IDUs had Hepatitis B
	CSW
	▓ Over 2,000 CSWs
	▓ Most originate from Moldova and Romania (higher HIV rate)
	International Workers and Peacekeeping Forces
	▓ 60,000–70,000 international workers
	▓ 17,500 international troops

Epidemiological Overview

Kosovo's health sector crumbled under the combined effects of neglect, ethnic disagreements, and chaos after the break-up of the former Yugoslavia. The legacy of these difficulties left a population with inadequate health coverage. The result is a deteriorated health status, limited access to health care for some populations, and a system that is heavily financed through out-of-pocket payments. There is concern that the negative effect of this status quo has fallen disproportionately on the most vulnerable groups in society. However, the absence of basic data systems makes health status measurement in post-conflict Kosovo especially difficult. Kosovo exhibits one of the lowest percentages of antenatal care for pregnant women and in births attended by a professional. According to the Bank's Poverty Assessment of 1999, 15 percent of pregnant women did not see a health care worker and 20 percent gave birth at home without professional help. The limited health data available suggest that Kosovo ranks lowest in Europe on almost every health indicator. Available data indicate that, even before the crisis, Kosovo had the poorest statistics in Europe on virtually every health indicator.

Donors responded generously to promote the reconstruction and recovery program in Kosovo. Overall, the emergency recovery and rehabilitation phase in Kosovo has essentially finished, with considerable achievements in all sectors. In terms of health, post-conflict reconstruction was concerned with the rebuilding of the health infrastructure and the establishment of institutional bodies to plan and manage it. The establishment of a Ministry of Health for the Provisional Self-Government in Kosovo in 2002, to replace the former Department of Health of the UNMIK administration, signaled the first steps in more local accountability for the Kosovo health sector following the initial period of stabilization.

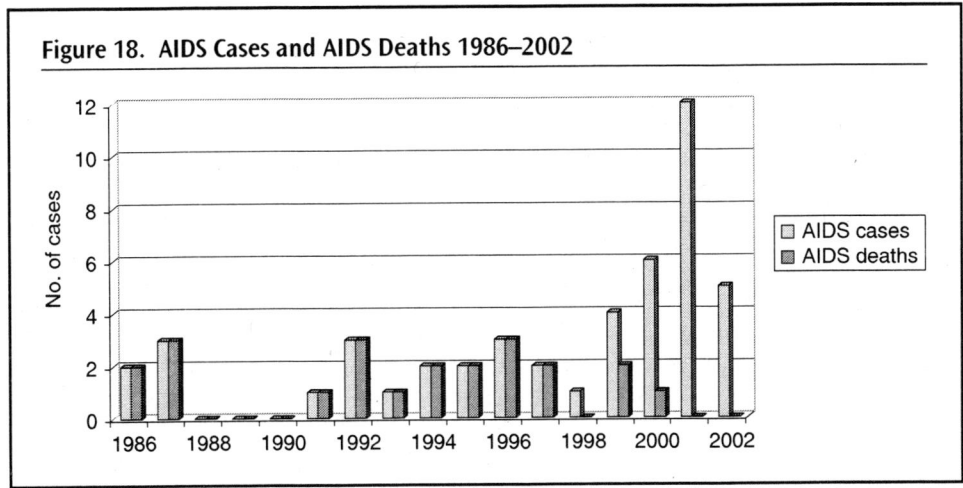

Figure 18. AIDS Cases and AIDS Deaths 1986–2002

Source: NIPH 2003.

HIV/AIDS

Existing data suggest that Kosovo is currently a low-prevalence, low-incidence region for HIV/AIDS infection. Notification data are shown in Figure 18. From 1986 to 2004, only 61 HIV/AIDS cases have been reported, having 25 already died. However, the number of reported cases increased in recent years after the war (12 in 2001 including 5 among foreigners). This increase may be partly due to improvements in reporting. The majority of AIDS patients were female (53 percent in the perido 1999–2004) and most were between

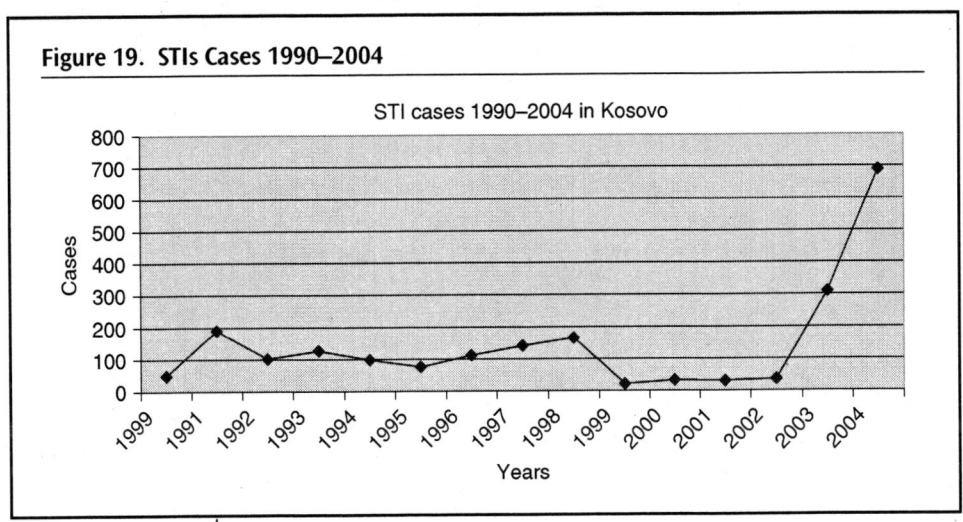

Figure 19. STIs Cases 1990–2004

Source: NIPH 2004.

the ages of 30 and 39. The main mode of HIV transmission is believed to be sexual contact, though there are no data to confirm this. From scarce data available from blood donors and patients tested at blood transfusion services, it is estimated that HIV prevalence is less than 0.1 percent. Since 1986, all blood donors have been tested for HIV, syphilis, and Hepatitis B and C. Four patients were tested positive for HIV out of the 1,776 outpatients tested in 2002, and 3 HIV positive patients out of the 856 outpatients tested in the first three months of 2003. Available data show that Hepatitis B among blood donors varied from about 3 to 7 percent; and prevalence of Hepatitis C was less than 0.2 percent. Researchers calculated the expected HIV prevalence in all TB patients in Kosovo to be between 0 and 3.6 percent. They concluded that if HIV prevalence is assumed to be six times greater in TB patients than in the general population, then HIV prevalence among Kosovo's general population may be estimated at 0 to 0.6 percent. [14]

Sexually-transmitted Infections

Accurate data about the number or types of STIs in Kosovo is not known. Although STIs are included in regular surveillance, reporting is unrealiable. During the 1990–2004 period, a total of 2,093 STI cases were reported by the Dermatological and Venereal Diseases Clinic. However, this is likely to be an underestimate, as two parallel systems were operating in Kosovo in the 1990s, and available figures do not represent the entire population. Approximately 80 percent of all diagnosed STI cases were from Priština. In 2001–2002, the Center for Blood Transfusion notified 6 positive cases of syphilis (TPHA), and 978 cases of Hepatitis B (HBV) cases. If the assays are working correctly, these data may suggest relatively low prevalence of syphilis infection in the population. A recent study conducted among outpatients attending a private gynecologic clinic in Priština ("Gynekos") during 2001–2002 paints a different picture of STI prevalence. During this period, 3 TPHA positive syphilis cases, 16 HIV positive cases, and 1,085 Hepatitis B positive cases were identified together with 1,100 cases of urethral discharge among men. Over two thousand females were diagnosed with vaginal or cervical discharge (Ferizi 2003). In addition, data reported by programs working with sex workers show very high prevalence of STIs among these women, especially of non-ulcerative STIs.

Vulnerability to HIV/AIDS: Contextual Factors

Kosovo's population is estimated at 2.4 million people. The Statistical Office of Kosovo estimates that 88 percent of the population is ethnic Kosovar Albanians. The ethnic Serbian population accounts for 7 percent of the population, followed by Bosniaks (1.9 percent), Roma

---

14. Researchers from the UNMIK Department of Health and Social Welfare, Columbia University, and Doctors of the World, interviewed patients (n = 98) between ages 18 and 60 in September 2001 who were currently on the TB wards of Priština University Hospital and four regional hospitals outside the capital. Participants were asked their age and if they had worked outside Kosovo for over one month. An OraQuick HIV 1–2 sample was obtained and developed. See Wennberg and Jakup (2002).

Table 60. Vulnerability Factors—Kosovo

GNI per Capita UNDP 2004	▧ 848 Euro
Unemployment MoFE	▧ 50% (63% among youth)
Poverty MoFE	▧ 15% in extreme poverty ($1/day)
Mobility	▧ 1.2 million Kosovars displaced internally or left Kosovo ▧ 900,000 people repatriated in 2002–2003
Trafficking	▧ Macedonia and Kosovo are primary transit and destination countries in the Balkans ▧ The lack of border control exacerbates the problem

(1.7 percent), and Turks (1 percent). Kosovo is predominantly Muslim (70 percent), followed by Eastern Orthodox (15 percent), Roman Catholic (4 percent), and Protestant (1 percent). The population is very young, with about one-third under 15 years of age and 57 percent under 25 years. Only about 6 percent of the population is 65 years and older. The dependency ratio is high, largely because of the large proportion of persons under age 15. There is a shortage of males ages 20 to 50 years, primarily caused by male emigration for economic reasons, leading to significantly more females than males in that age group. Kosovo is divided into 30 municipalities. According to the EU, about two-thirds of Kosovo's population lives in 1,500 villages, with only nine urban areas having over 20,000 inhabitants. A large diaspora, primarily in Western Europe, plays an important role in Kosovo's economy through remittances and the financing of parallel structures developed throughout the 1990s (Statistical Office of Kosovo 2003a; EC and The World Bank 2003).

Albanian and Serb communities remain largely separated and up to 200,000 people remain displaced—although 2003 did see many ethnic Serbs return to their homes in Kosovo, partly encouraged by programs for returnees for which the Government provided $10 million in 2003. The extreme poverty and lack of social integration of the Roma population also remains an issue, although the number of Roma in Kosovo is proportionately smaller than in Macedonia, Montenegro and Serbia.

Economy

After significant economic declines in the late-1990s, growth bounced back immediately after the end of the conflict. The adoption of the Deutsche Mark, and subsequently the Euro, as well as the maintenance of a liberal trade regime has resulted in a relatively high degree of macro-economic stability in Kosovo. As common in many post-conflict environments, Kosovo experienced robust, double-digit growth rates in 2000 and 2001. This has resulted in average GDP per capita doubling from less than $400 in 2000 to about $640 in 2002 and almost US$790 in 2003.[15] Growth has, however, begun to slow down. Growth has also been especially driven by a large number of new small and medium enterprises (SMEs) concentrated in the construction, service, and retailing sectors, especially catering to the international community in and around Priština. Small-scale agricultural production has also rebounded and provides employment for two-thirds of the population, who live in rural areas. Growth has also been dependent on generous donor assistance for reconstruction and on remittances from the Kosovo diaspora.

Poverty

Kosovo was traditionally the poorest province in the Socialist Federal Republic of Yugoslavia (EC and the World Bank 2003; U.S. Department of State 2003d). Despite initial progress in reconstruction and economic recovery, poverty remains widespread. Four years after the end of the conflict, Kosovo remains the poorest area in Europe, with persistent and widespread poverty. Average incomes rebounded strongly after the cessation of hostilities, but incomes are still well below pre-conflict levels. About 36 percent of the population lives below the poverty line. Poverty is especially concentrated among non-Albanian ethnic groups and there are large gender inequalities.

While less common, extreme poverty remains a major problem. About 15 percent of the population lives below the extreme (food) poverty line of 0.93 per day. There is a strong correlation between extreme poverty and those people who are landless, have little formal education, have large numbers of children, or are disabled. Gender and ethnicity also have important correlations with extreme poverty; further there is a relatively high incidence of extreme poverty among female-headed households and among the non-Albanian and Serb ethnic groups (especially the Roma, the Muslim Slav, and the Gorani). Extreme poverty also has a strong regional dimension. According to UNDP Human Developemnt Index, the highest levels of poverty are found in Shtime, Gllogoc/Drenas, Deçan, Kaçanik, Malishevë. Finally, extreme poverty appears more pronounced in secondary cities than in rural areas or in the capital city.

Unemployment is a particular concern in Kosovo and is closely linked to poverty. Official estimates indicate that 49 percent of the workforce is not formally employed—although many of these people are engaged in subsistence farming or the informal economy. Hence, more detailed analysis suggests that the number of people looking for employment is between 20–30 percent and many of these are long-term unemployed. Unemployment is also a particular problem among youth, with large numbers of new job seekers entering the workforce each year.

---

15. All economic statistics in Kosovo are subject to a considerable degree of uncertainty. There has not been a reliable census in Kosovo for two decades. GNI figures are especially subject to a very high degree of uncertainty as they are based on assumptions and hypotheses regarding capital flows from seasonal workers temporarily residing abroad. Latest estimates are based on considerable work during 2003 by the Ministry of Finance and Economy, supported by the IMF and the Bank. Recent estimates suggest that the economy may not be as large as previously thought, but show a consistent pattern of strong growth immediately after the conflict, supported by generous donor flows.

Mobility

There has been a massive movement of people in Kosovo, but no census has been carried out after the conflict. During the conflict, over 1.2 million Kosovars were internally displaced or left Kosovo; by mid-2003, over 900,000 had returned (IOM and UNICEF 2002). Most of the refugees went to neighboring countries. It is estimated that over 800,000 Kosovar Albanians fled to neighboring Albania, Bosnia and Herzegovina, Macedonia and other parts of FRY, plus tens of thousands fled to other countries during the course of the conflict. More than half a million were internally displaced and over 12,000 were killed. Over 100,000 ethnic Serbs had also fled Kosovo by the end of the hostilities. With this exodus, many institutions lost their staffing and management. While by late August 1999, most Kosovar Albanian refugees had returned, the post-conflict period has seen a massive exodus of Serb Kosovars, with the consequent loss of vital technical and managerial skills in administration and public enterprises. Many Kosovars are now restricted from traveling to other countries due to difficulties in obtaining visas. In 2001, the conflict in Macedonia resulted in an influx of about 80,000 refugees into Kosovo. Though limited in duration, this inflow had a severe impact on local Kosovar communities, especially on those bordering Macedonia (EC and The World Bank 2003). Refugees International highlights that despite the influx of refugees, the region remains unequipped to provide shelter and basic social welfare programs (Refugees International 2003).

Vulnerable Groups

Although HIV prevalence is low, Kosovo has identifiable factors that put the population at risk. These factors include having a large young population, high unemployment, high levels of mobility of Kosovars in and out of the region, rapid social changes, a growing drug problem and commercial sex industry, a highly stigmatized MSM population, and the presence of an international community.

Youth. More than half (57 percent) of Kosovo's population is under the age of 25. The majority of young people in Kosovo have been affected by years of oppression and increasing violence, with many having been forced from their homes (IOM and UNICEF 2002). The 1999 LSMS found large inequalities in education across income, ethnicity, and gender. Although net enrollment rates in primary school are on average high (97 percent), only 76 percent of children under 14 from ethnic groups other than Serbs and Albanians are enrolled in school. Gender inequality in secondary school enrollment is even more dramatic; just over half of Albanian girls ages 15–18 were enrolled in school in 2000, compared to nearly 75 percent of Albanian boys. According to UNFPA, 10 percent of Kosovar females are illiterate, compared to only 2.3 percent of males. Net enrollment rates in secondary education for other ethnic groups are on average less than 55 percent. Youth from the poorest deciles in rural areas are less than half as likely to enroll in secondary education than their counterparts in the top decile. Economic factors are the main correlates of non-enrollment. Nearly all households with children enrolled in the academic year prior to the survey (99 percent) made considerable out-of-pocket payments. Geographic and ethnic differences are also evident, with expenditure higher in urban areas, particularly for Serbs. Safety, as well as access to schools (especially in rural areas), is also identified as barriers to enrollment.

International Workers and Peacekeeping Forces. Many international organizations are present in Kosovo—there are approximately 60,000 to 70,000 international workers in Kosovo. Large international peacekeeping forces are also present in Kosovo, rotating after an average stay of six months. However, during 2003, KFOR was gradually reduced to 17,500 international troops, down from over 50,000 international troops in 1999. The UNMIK clinic deals with HIV cases and is responsible for decisions related to medical repatriation. Although some KFOR troops are provided HIV/AIDS education (primarily related to condom distribution and use), few international organizations provide adequate HIV/AIDS interventions for their staff. Population Services International's peer education project is working with the Kosovo military (IOM and UNICEF 2002). In 2001, a Joint Military Civil Alliance mission to Kosovo noted that the introduction of a large number of foreign officers and staff had a significant influence, both positive and negative, on local social and economic dynamics. The mission highlighted areas requiring improvement, including an assessment of the impact of peacekeeping operations on HIV/AIDS and an assessment of peacekeeper training related to gender issues, professional conduct, and STI prevention to ensure a more coordinated response (UNAIDS 2001b).

Sex Workers and Trafficking. As is the case in neighboring countries, accurate information on the sex industry is lacking, but it is estimated that at least 2,000 women are engaged in commercial sex work (CSW). According to the International Organization for Migration and UNICEF, the Kosovar conflict exacerbated and increased trafficking of women for sexual exploitation into Kosovo. Macedonia and Kosovo are primary transit and destination countries. The majority of CSWs originate from Moldova and Romania, which have a higher HIV prevalence. Internal trafficking cases are increasingly reported within Kosovo and Albania. As commercial sex work is illegal in Kosovo, much of the prostitution has gone underground, which has made it extremely difficult to reach CSWs. Therefore, no data are available regarding HIV prevalence, risk behaviors, or related knowledge among sex workers (IOM and UNICEF 2002).

The Special Representative of the UN Secretary General introduced a trafficking regulation with the force of law in 2001; the Trafficking and Prostitution Investigation Unit, comprising UN police and Kosovo Police Service officers, is charged with enforcing the regulation (U.S. Department of State 2003d). According to the EU, Kosovo is facing an increase in local and regional crime. The lack of specialized local border personnel and effective judicial administration systems impede Kosovos's ability to respond effectively to crime. In Kosovo, policing is a shared responsibility between the United Nations Civilian Police (CIVPOL) and the Kosovo Police Service (EuropeAid 2003a).

According to UNIFEM, the Kosovo conflict had devastating effects on women and girls in general. During 1998–1999, many women lost family members, became victims of brutal violence, and endured intense insecurity and fear. For women, the exodus to neighboring countries, lengthy stays in refugee camps, and widespread displacement in other countries had particularly difficult implications, compounded by the pressure of caring for nuclear and extended families. Women have continued to face multiple losses of family and property. Following the deaths of their spouses, some women became the only breadwinners in their families. Kosovar women continue to face issues regarding human rights, illiteracy, access to education, unemployment, and lack of social services, high birth rates, high maternal mortality, domestic violence, and trafficking. Minority women suffer from restrictions of movement, insecurity about the future, unemployment, and persistent fear of violence throughout their communities (Ástgeirsdóttir 2001).

MSM. There is little information available on homosexuality or men having sex with men (MSM) in Kosovo. Similar to other countries in the region, there is a strong stigma regarding MSM, such that the MSM community is largely underground (IOM and UNICEF 2002). According to anecdotal data, it appears that MSM have limited knowledge about the risks of unprotected sex and that use of condoms is low. In early 2003, the first local gay NGO was established, although it is not yet officially registered.

Drug Users. Kosovo is a key transit route for heroin into Europe, and there may be as many as 5,000 heroin users in the region at the present time. Information describing the extent and patterns of drug use in Kosovo is thin. However, a WHO/UNICEF Rapid Assessment (RAR) carried out in 2001 suggests that, although injecting drug use is limited, there is rapid growth in the practice, with heroin being the main drug of use. Among young people attending school, levels of drug use (alcohol, tobacco, and other drugs) were comparable with most EU countries, but levels of heroin use among young adults were slightly higher. Among young adults, there were comparatively few IDUs, although there is evidence that young users are increasingly injecting. Increases in heroine users are thought to have resulted from increases in drug supply, as well as changes in local patterns of production and consumption, increased travel, migration, and cross-border trade. Sharing of needles among IDUs is very common. All 20 hospitalized IDUs had Hepatitis B. The combination of drug users sharing injecting equipment and use of drugs that impact sexual behavior is significantly increasing the likelihood of contracting HIV.

Prisoners. The prison centers in Kosovo are under the management of UNMIK Department of Justice-Penal Management Division. The penal system includes eight prisons and detention centers located around Kosovo with over 1,000 prisoners. Health care is available for prisoners through the Department of Justice. No routine evaluation or screening of STIs or HIV is in place.

HIV/AIDS Awareness and Knowledge

A Knowledge, Attitude and Practice (KAP) study in 2000, and a KAP household survey in 2003[16] revealed that knowledge of HIV and STIs among Kosovars was low, and that people who were HIV positive were highly stigmatized. The IPH survey found that only 12 percent of respondents had correct information regarding HIV transmission. There was also limited knowledge about other STIs. Many people did not think they were at high risk of HIV infection. Knowledge about modes of transmission was higher than knowledge about correct ways of protection against the infection. Young women know about condoms, but most view condoms as a means of contraception rather than a method to prevent disease.

---

16. Surveys on knowledge, attitudes, and practices regarding HIV/AIDS/STIs were conducted by the Institute for Public Health (IPH) in Priština in 2000 (with support from WHO) and Population Services International in 2001 (with support from UNFPA and UNICEF), and 2003. The IPH survey was conducted among those ages 14 to 19 years (n = 209). The PSI survey was carried out among 15- to 49-year-olds (n = 2,256).

Table 61. Knowledge, Attitudes, and Practices—Kosovo

KAP	General population
KAP Study 2000 Household survey 2003	▓ 12% had correct information about HIV transmission
	▓ Condoms viewed mostly as a method of contraception
	▓ Condoms are distributed by local NGOs
	Kosovar youth age 15–25 years
	▓ 80% knew that condoms and abstinence reduce risk of HIV/AIDS
	▓ 25% believe that condoms do not protect against HIV/STIs
	▓ 50% use condoms always or most of time, mostly for preventing unwanted pregnancy

Approximately 80 percent of respondents reported that they would demand an HIV-infected person be removed from their class, and only 11 percent would continue a friendship with an HIV-positive person. One-quarter of respondents believed that condoms do not protect them against HIV and STIs (IOM and UNICEF 2002). However, the household survey in 2003, performed among Kosovar ages 15 to 25 indicated that young people had gained more knowledge about HIV/AIDS and its prevention as a result of various campaigns carried out by MOH in cooperation with NGOs. Among the respondents to this survey, all had heard about the risk of HIV, and 80 percent knew that abstinence and condoms could reduce the risk of transmitting HIV/AIDS. Less than half of the sample reported having had sex, but of those, only half use a condom always or most of the time, mostly for limiting pregnancy.

Governance

Kosovo's final status remains uncertain, and a UN interim administration continues to be the final authority. On June 10, 1999, the United Nations Security Council adopted Resolution 1244 (UNSCR 1244), which provides the legal framework for Kosovo's current status. Until a political solution to the Kosovo crisis can be found, UNSCR 1244 affirmed the sovereignty and territorial integrity of Serbia and Montenegro (SAM) but also called for 'substantial autonomy' for Kosovo. UNSCR 1244 authorized the establishment of "an international civil presence in Kosovo in order to provide an interim administration" which has been implemented through the creation of the United Nations Mission in Kosovo (UNMIK). Progress toward self-government in Kosovo is continuing. The adoption of the Constitutional Framework in May 2001 signaled a key step in the transition to self-government. The Provisional Institutions of Self-Government (PISG) comprise the President of Kosovo; a 120 member Assembly; and an Executive branch that is headed by a Prime Minister and a Cabinet of 10 Ministers. The Provincial Institutions of Self-Government (PISG) has significant responsibility for governing Kosovo, although the UN retains final legal authority and certain reserve powers. The final batch of responsibilities was formally transferred to the PISG on December 30, 2003.

Since 2001, democracy, the rule of law, human rights, and engagement of civil society have improved. Two local elections to municipal assemblies have been successfully undertaken;

power has been decentralized to local government; there is a gradual shift in administration mandates from international to local actors; and security has improved with the 1999 creation of the Kosovo Police Service (EuropeAid 2003a). However, challenges include strengthening the institutional capacity of the Assembly, along with that of central and local government; greater transfer of responsibilities to local actors; further development of civil society; and combating organized crime. The situation for ethnic minorities remains very difficult. For example, minority communities in specific locations have little real access to banks, business and social services, or mainstream EU assistance interventions. Violence against Kosovar minorities has increased and became more organized (Refugees International 2003).

According to a 2003 report by the U.S.-based Management Systems International prepared for USAID, despite public opinion and discussions in the mass media that presume very high levels of public corruption, corruption does not appear to be a pervasive force in the governance process nor does it appear to undermine significantly the capacity of the Government to perform its duties. Other findings suggest that if economic stagnation continues, the impact of even the most effective governance reform and law enforcement programs against corruption are not likely to prevent corrupt practices (Spector, Winbourne, andd Beck 2003).

Health Care in Kosovo

Kosovo has a tradition of a publicly provided health care system financed through social health insurance. Until 1989, the system was typical of those in Eastern European countries, which were dominated by large policlinics and hospitals. From 1989, the health system suffered a significant decline. Large sections of the population were excluded from using the system. Consequently, they became dependent on a parallel network of services provided by NGOs, they paid for health care out of pocket, or it was provided to them on a voluntary basis. Post-conflict reconstruction has been concerned with the rebuilding of the health sector and the establishment of institutional bodies to plan and manage it. The establishment of a Ministry of Health for the Provisional Self-Government in Kosovo in 2002, to replace the former Department of Health of the UNMIK administration, signaled the first steps in more local accountability for the Kosovo health sector following the initial period of stabilization.

According to the draft 2004 Poverty Assessment, in general, the provision of health services is quantitatively reasonable in Kosovo, but some important barriers to access exist, particularly for the poorest, the elderly, and the disabled. The health services network, both at primary health care (PHC) and secondary/tertiary care levels, is quantitatively adequate and geographically well distributed. However, in some cases, there is a lack of medical and nursing staff to ensure effective accessibility during the day to PHC services. In addition, a limited number of areas need better infrastructure for tertiary care, including equipment and training. The main barriers to access to health services include, inter alia: (i) limited functioning of PHC in rural areas; (ii) costs—including informal payments and drugs that should be provided by the system, but are not; (iii) lack of confidence by the public in the health system, particularly at the primary level. In principle, health facilities are accessible to everybody regardless of ethnicity. MOH supports a few small hospitals and health facilities run by Serbian health personnel. However, most of the Kosovar Serbs utilize a parallel health system directly subsidized by Serbia and Montenegro, which does not report to MOH.

With support from EAR, MOH has been implementing two- and three-year training programs for family doctors. As of the end of April 2004, more than 400 physicians have received this training. In addition, with support from Finland, training for family medicine nurses is being provided. One important achievement of the physicians training is that the program was accredited by the Royal College of Physicians of the UK. However, changes in the organizational model of primary health care are yet to be developed to ensure that the principles of the family medicine model are implemented in the PHC. The Primary Health Care Services are provided through a network of health houses and ambulantas (280 facilities). The health houses provide the traditional PHC services, including general practice, pediatric, obstetric, and dental services and also, in some cases, a range of specialized health care services. In 2002, responsibility for the provision of primary care services was devolved to the municipalities. Kosovo has a relatively modest level of public inpatient hospital provision, about 5,000 beds or 2.3 beds per 1,000 people. Performance of the hospital sector is weak with length of stay relatively long (10.6 days in 2001) and average occupancy low (68 percent in 2001).

In theory, everyone living in Kosovo is entitled to free access to basic health care services, but the reality is quite different (Goodson 2003). Barriers to access are the result, in part, of the systematic discrimination of the Albanian minority in the former Yugoslavia throughout the 1990s. Poor access to health care is a particular problem for women and children. Another common barrier to health care in Kosovo is the cost of the service. It is reported that currently over 95 percent of the population pays for health service, independent of whether it is provided in public or private facilities. As per the LSMS data from 2001, an average of 28 percent of people who reported a medical problem for which they did not seek treatment could not afford health care. This percentage increases to nearly 33 percent for the prime age cohort (age 25–49). Unsurprisingly, financial considerations when seeking health care seem to be more binding for the individuals in the bottom two consumption deciles. Another common barrier to access, especially in rural areas, is the distance to the facility.

Funding of Health Services

As part of the former Yugoslav Republic, the health system was financed through a social health insurance system. In the years leading up to the war, the systems began to decay and many of the Albanian population were excluded. Since 1999, when UNMIK assumed responsibility for the health system, financing has been undertaken by a combination of public finance from general taxation through the Kosovo Consolidated Budget, personal contributions, and donor support. In 2002, a VAT and payroll taxation was introduced. Personal and private expenditure on health is a significant factor in financing health care services, including a combination of formal co-payments, fees paid to the private sector, and informal payments to professionals in public health care institutions.

Public health expenditures are relatively low. According to Government estimates, in 2003, public health expenditures were 4.4 percent of GDP, which is below the regional averages and well below the neighbor countries with the exception of Albania. Prospects

Table 62. Estimated Costs of HIV/AIDS Activities in Kosovo (US$ Thousands)

	2001	2002	2003	2004	2005	2006	2007
Prevention	1,008	1,324	1,647	1,979	2,320	2,670	3,028
Youth	24	27	31	34	37	40	43
CSW	16	30	47	66	89	114	143
MSMs	45	77	111	147	185	225	266
IDU	3	5	7	9	12	14	16
Condom social marketing	4	34	63	93	123	153	183
Condom provision	11	84	158	232	308	386	464
STI management	49	84	122	162	203	246	289
VCT	1	6	10	14	19	23	28
Workplace	50	84	119	155	192	231	270
Blood Safety	310	313	316	318	321	324	326
PMTCT	5	8	10	13	15	18	21
Mass media	490	571	653	734	816	898	979
Treatment	28	57	101	180	301	478	718
Palliative care	5	8	11	15	19	23	27
Testing	0	0	0	0	0	0	0
OI Treatment	20	34	46	62	80	100	124
OI Prevention	2	4	7	12	20	31	45
Lab HAART	1	5	16	38	76	134	216
ARV	1	7	22	54	107	190	306
Policy, advocacy, administration and research	52	69	87	108	131	157	187
TOTAL	1,036	1,381	1,749	2,159	2,621	3,148	3,746

for 2003–2005 are for a very small increase of public expenditure in absolute terms (less than 5 percent in three years).

Allocation of funds to fight and prevent infectious diseases, including HIV/AIDS, is limited. However, the MOH provided funds for the Kosovo AIDS Office in 2002 and the 2003 budget includes funding for HIV/AIDS treatment. The MOH and international donors have all made a commitment to funding HIV/AIDS prevention programs and the development of the HIV/AIDS Strategic Plan. UNAIDS and other organizations support the early implementation of programs. The Kosovo AIDS Committee has estimated that it would need about $10 million for the period 2005–2007 (Table 62).

Government and Civil Society Action on HIV/AIDS

The HIV/AIDS Strategic, Policy, and Regulatory Framework

Despite the difficult conditions described above, interim authorities and the new elected administration have made HIV/AIDS a priority in the health sector. The recently adopted

Table 63. Government Intervention and Institutional Arrangements—Kosovo	
Intersectoral coordination	▨ Kosovo AIDS Committee established in 2000
	▨ InterMinisterial Commission for Psychoactive Substances for Implementation of RAR recommendations established
	▨ Prime Minister's Office established Interministerial Group for Anti-Trafficking Issues
National HIV/AIDS Strategy and Legislation	▨ Health Policy Guidelines for Kosovo address five priorities for health care including reducing HIV/AIDS
	▨ Action Plan for the Establishment of a Comprehensive HIV/AIDS Prevention Program for Kosovo issued by KAC 2001
	▨ Kosovo Strategy for HIV/AIDS for 2004–2008 was approved in 2003
	▨ GFATM proposal prepared by CCM
Government institution responsible for HIV/AIDS	▨ Kosovo AIDS Committee (KAC) established in 2000
	▨ Trafficking and Prostitution Investigation Unit created by the Special representative of UN Secretary General in 2001

Health Policy Guidelines for Kosovo address five priorities for health care: (i) healthy start in life; (ii) improving health of young people; (iii) improving mental health; (iv) developing human resources for health; and (v) reducing communicable diseases, including HIV/AIDS. A short-term action plan for HIV/AIDS had been prepared in 2001 by the Kosovo AIDS Committee (KAC), but due to lack of funding, the plan was never implemented. The MOH and KAC organized a strategic planning workshop in September 2002 to initiate the development of the Kosovo Strategy for HIV/AIDS for 2004–2008, which was approved in 2004; and established three Technical Working Groups (TWG). These groups include representatives from the Ministries of Health; Youth, Sport and Culture; Education, Science and Technology; Kosovo Protection Corps (KPC); Kosovo Police Service (KPS); NGOs; and international donors. Development of the strategy was coordinated by the HIV/AIDS office of the Ministry of Health. This work was co-financed by USAID, the European Agency for Reconstruction, the Canadian International Development Agency, and other stakeholders. Kosovo submitted a grant proposal to the Global Fund to Fight AIDs, TB and Malaria, which however was not not approved, but the CCM was encouraged to apply again.

The five-year strategic HIV/AIDS action plan will facilitate the development of cost-effective programs and their implementation, monitoring, and evaluation, as well as the mobilization of the needed resources. The plan focuses on:

▨ Legislation.
▨ HIV/AIDS prevention in vulnerable population groups: young people, men who have sex with men, commercial sex workers and their clients, drug users, prisoners.
▨ Health personnel and law enforcement: improving the occupational safety of health personnel to reduce risk of exposure to HIV/AIDS; involving law enforcement agencies in reaching vulnerable groups.
▨ Surveillance system: establishment of a systematic and comprehensive STI–HIV/AIDS surveillance system.

■ Testing, treatment, care, and follow-up services: establishment of voluntary coun-seling and testing, treatment (including post exposure prophylaxis care) and follow-up services.

An Inter-Ministerial Commission on Psychoactive Substances (IMCPS) was established is 2001. The current and new draft of the criminal code do not criminalize the use of drugs or possession of drugs for personal consumption. An important element of the current draft code is the differentiation between drug dealing and trafficking on one hand, and the use and possession of drugs for own consumption on the other. The Commission com-prises officials from the ministries concerned with youth, education, culture, social wel-fare, health, police, and criminal justice. There is a growing momentum within the Government to develop and implement a sound drug policy that would include harm reduction for HIV/AIDS.

Monitoring and evaluation of HIV/AIDS and STIs activities in Kosovo has to be devel-oped, which requires financial and technical support.

Table 64. Government Intervention and Institutional Arrangements—Kosovo

Testing	■ Laboratory support is very limited and ELISA is not widely available
	■ Voluntary HIV tests offered by several laboratories
	■ Voluntary testing done through CID and sent to Pristina University Clinical Center
	■ Some STIs and HIV diagnostics are available at KFOR and UNMIK Health Clinic
	■ No Counseling provided
Surveillance	■ The system is very weak but emphasis is on high-risk groups
	■ Sentinel sites for HIV/AIDS established but functioning poorly
	■ Institute for Public Health in Pristina conducted KAP survey on HIV/AIDS in 2000 with support from WHO
HIV/AIDS Notification	■ National IPH receives information on all registered HIV/ADS cases
Blood Safety	■ Blood donors tested for HIV, syphilis and Hepatitis B and C since 1986
	■ Donated Blood is screened using quick test method
	■ Blood donated mostly from family members
	■ Donated blood is sent to Blood Transfusion Unit, Pristina University Clinical Center
Prevention	■ HIV/AIDS prevention among vulnerable groups and health staff are important part of 5 year strategic plan prepared by KAC and MOH
	■ Peer educators training on prevention of HIV/AIDS and sexual reproductive health conducted by UNICEF
	■ Multiple other preventive projects targeting IDU and condom use are implemented by NGO sector
Treatment	■ HIV AIDS patients are treated at the Clinic for Infectious disease of the University Clinic Center in Pristina
	■ There are no OI drugs and ARVs available through the public health system

Surveillance of HIV/AIDS and STIs

The current surveillance system in Kosovo for HIV and STIs is very weak or almost non-existent and, therefore, data on incidence and prevalence are quite limited. HIV screening of all blood donations is mandatory and becomes a source of data for the surveillance system. From 1990–2002, 1,095 STI cases were reported. However, this is likely to be an underestimate because two parallel systems operated in Kosovo during that period, and available figures do not represent the entire population. Although the national IPH should receive reports of all STIs, the system is clearly not functioning well. Many Kosovars are treated for STIs in private health clinics, but no system of reporting by the private sector is currently in place. Kosovo does not report data on HIV infections nor AIDS cases to the European Center for the Epidemiological Monitoring of AIDS (EuroHIV 2003).

However, faced with the fast developing epidemic in other countries in the region, the IPH and the HIV/AIDS Office in collaboration with international institutions and NGOs are committed to establishing a Kosovar STIs and HIV/AIDS Surveillance Plan. This plan is a follow-up to the Action Plan for the Establishment of a Comprehensive HIV/AIDS Prevention Program for Kosovo issued in 2001. Because of the low prevalence characteristics, the emphasis is placed on those groups where the epidemic started developing in neighboring countries: IDUs, CSWs, and MSM. Training in STI—HIV surveillance and epidemiology is planned for the staff, especially pertaining to high-risk groups. Routine surveillance of STIs was initiated in 2000 and requires reporting of three STI syndromes (vaginal and urethral discharge, and genital ulcers). No biological prevalence studies have been conducted on STIs. The current program to establish sentinel sites for STIs and HIV/AIDS surveillance found that the present data collection systems are functioning poorly; further there is a lack of treatment guidelines and information on high risk groups and vulnerable populations.

The Priština Clinical University Center Blood Transfusion Unit tests donated blood for HIV, syphilis, and Hepatitis B and C (UNFPA 2003b). Blood is also similarly tested in areas outside Priština, but quality control is a major concern. No official accreditation program for STIs and HIV testing currently exists. Voluntary HIV tests are available through the Clinic for Infectious Diseases of the University Clinical Center in Priština, where blood is collected; it is then sent to the Priština Clinical University Center Blood Transfusion Unit for testing. However, confidentiality is not ensured, and no pre- or post-test counseling by trained counselors is provided. HIV testing and counseling are conducted as part of training programs for VCT at three selected sites (Regional Institute of Public Health in Prizren, Infective Clinic PUH, and private lab "Bioticus" in Priština) using rapid tests. HIV testing is available for troops of the American and French KFOR contingents, and the IOM conducts HIV testing on a regular basis to assess the health of immigration applicants (IOM and UNICEF 2002). There are essentially no youth-friendly testing services in Kosovo.

Laboratory support for STI diagnosis is very limited: recognized standards are not always met, and limited and inconsistent availability of supplies reduces usefulness of the available equipment. In most cases, diagnoses are made based on direct microscope observation, cultures, some latex tests and, more recently, ELISA for HIV. Some STI and HIV diagnostics are available at British KFOR, Main KFOR, U.S. KFOR, and UNMIK Health Clinic. Also, in the central laboratory at IPH, some space has been allocated for the development of STI laboratory work. A laboratory for genito-urinary infections exists within the Department of Microbiology at the National Institute of Public Health, but a separate laboratory for STI does not exist. The majority of patients are, therefore, treated syndromically. However, it is uncertain to what extent this syndromic management conforms to WHO guidelines. Many Kosovars seek STI treatment within the private health sector, and there are currently no screening programs to identify asymptomatic individuals. It is possible that patients go directly to pharmacies and acquire medication without prescriptions.

HIV/AIDS and STIs Prevention and Control in the Public System

Much work has yet to be done to achieve a new level of knowledge and safe practices in young people and other vulnerable groups in Kosovo. Many activities conducted since 1999 have predominately focused on increasing knowledge about HIV/AIDS and promoting prevention messages among the general population. The International Medical Corps (IMC) has established five youth centers in the largest urban centers outside Priština. They focus on young people (ages 15–24) and provide group and individual counseling, addressing life skills and sexuality. IMC offers condom demonstrations, but this remains a sensitive subject especially for young people.

The RAR (IOM and UNICEF 2002) found that HIV/AIDS prevention interventions have been impeded by the lack of an overall policy for dealing with existing and potential drug-related problems, as well as a lack of coordination at both policy and implementation level. Providing adequate assistance is also hampered by the general absence of outreach and prevention services targeted to drug users, especially vulnerable young people, and by the absence of harm reduction services. The RAR recommended that action focus on:

- Policy development and coordination: aimed at identifying the major issues regarding substance abuse problems, formulating strategies, allocating a budget, and defining a structure for coordinating and supporting policy implementation.
- Primary prevention: aimed at information/education/awareness activities.
- Secondary prevention: including professional treatment and support services.
- Tertiary prevention: including harm reduction and activities aimed at preventing transmission of blood-borne viruses via unhygienic syringes.
- Monitoring and research.

Primary prevention has begun through support to health education in schools and in the university for students, as well as general messages through posters and other media. University students are provided with education on STIs by the staff at the university health center. All regional IPHs have a designated staff member responsible for health promotion and health education activities, including teaching students at secondary schools. Municipalities are expected to participate in prevention work, and allocate funding for these activities.

HIV/AIDS and STIs Treatment in the Public System

Treatment for IDUs is available only at the Neuropsychiatry Department of the University Clinical Center and a private clinic in Priština, but no methadone therapy is available. HIV/AIDS patients are treated at the Clinic for Infectious Diseases of the University Clinical Center in Priština. Treatment of opportunistic infections and HIV/AIDS was not available in the public health system (IOM and UNICEF 2002), but in 2005 the Govenrment started OI and ARV drugs. There are no specialized STI clinics except the tertiary-level specialized dermatovenereological clinic in Kosovo. No special training on STIs exists outside the regular Medical School curriculum or residency. STI services are provided as a part of other health services through gynecologists, urologists, and dermatovenereologists in major regional medical centers and through primary care structures elsewhere.

HIV/AIDS Prevention and Control by NGOs

In 2002, over 50 civil society groups and NGOs received EU support, totaling €4.3 million, through the Kosovo Civil Society Foundation. Grants support initiatives including the participation of women in politics, capacity building and training in project management, minority rights, computer classes for the Roma community, and youth networking activities. A minority fund has also been established to address the socioeconomic needs of minority communities in Kosovo. However, since the first AIDS case was registered in 1986, little work has been done with drug users, sex workers, MSM, and mobile populations.

Information on work by other NGOs on HIV/AIDS is listed below (IOM and UNICEF 2002).

Table 65. NGO Sector in Kosovo

▦ Over 50 civil society groups and NGOs received EU support totaling 4.3 million Euro in 2002.

▦ The Kosovo Protection Corps (KPC) was established in September 1999 as part of the Kosovo Liberation Army's transformation into a civilian, multidisciplinary, and multiethnic civil protection organization. It has a medical unit with a staff of 289 throughout the region, but only one infectious disease specialist among them. KPC appears to be eager to support initiatives of WHO and other international organizations in HIV/AIDS prevention, but is hampered by limited funds.

▦ Children's Aid Direct provides peer education and formal education on HIV/AIDS prevention through youth centers.

▦ PSI has been active in Kosovo since September 2000. It has four projects focusing on HIV/AIDS in the province. First, following formative research, PSI produced two television pieces promoting condom use and advising people of risks of HIV. Second, PSI's peer-to-peer youth project trained 150 adolescent peer educators in HIV/AIDS and STI prevention and issues surrounding unplanned pregnancy. Trained outreach workers have presented this information to about 6,500 secondary school students in Priština (over half of all secondary students in Priština). The peer education project will expand to all larger towns in Kosovo. It will also expand to include sex workers, IDUs, and MSM. Third, PSI has conducted training for activists and health educators on how to advocate for better reproductive health, with a focus on HIV/AIDS prevention. Fourth, to remove some of the barriers to healthier behavior, PSI is socially marketing the condom Love Plus.

▦ The United Methodist Committee on Relief launched a project in July 2002 that seeks to increase access to quality sexual health services for bartenders/sex workers. Ten private gynecologists throughout Kosovo were selected to participate in the project.

▦ The American Red Cross and the International Federation of Red Cross and Red Crescent Societies have partnered with the local Red Cross in Kosovo to establish the Community Resource Center Initiative. The Community Resource Centers provide counseling; support groups for women, children and families of the missing; health education; community-building activities; relief distributions; and referral services for psychological support and legal assistance.

Table 66. World Bank Support—Kosovo

Projects that address HIV directly	Projects that could include HIV/AIDS action	Analytical work that addresses HIV or some of the risk factors
Kosovo Youth Grant	Social Protection	
	Education Participation Improvement	
	Kosovo Education and Health Community Development Fund	

International Partner Organizations

The donor community provides extensive support to Kosovo, but this support is rapidly diminishing. Until 2002, donor assistance focused primarily on rehabilitation of the physical infrastructure in Kosovo. There is now an increasing emphasis on good governance, the rule of law, and developing the institutional capacity and legal frameworks for sustained socioeconomic development (EuropeAid 2003; IOM and UNICEF 2002). Some information on HIV-related work by international organizations is listed below.

Table 67. International Support—Kosovo

UN-TG	HIV prevention among CSW, funded by the UNAIDS PAF up to the end of 2005.
	HIV prevention among IDU.
	Establishment of the M&E unit inside the Kosovo AIDS Committee.
	HIV/AIDS Surveillance Unit at the National Institute of Public Health of Kosovo for the establishment of the HIV sentinel sites (June 2005).
	HIV/AIDS Adviser to the Office of AIDS in the Ministry of Health, acting also as UNTG Focal Point for Kosovo (Ended at 15 of March 2005).
UNICEF	Provides TA and capacity building to Kosovo HIV/AIDS Committee.
	Provides peer educators training on prevention of HIV/AIDS and sexual reproductive health.
	Supports awareness-raising and social mobilization activities on risks and prevention of HIV/AIDS/STIs.
	Involved in information and training projects, including the publication of a youth journal, inclusion of healthy lifestyle activities in school curricula, and development of a communication strategy.
	Undertakes awareness raising activities on child rights and trafficking among children and young people.
	Assists with development of legal and policy framework for juveniles in conflict with the law.
	Supports UNMIK's Victim Advocacy and Assistance Unit, Department of Justice.
	Undertook a rapid appraisal review (RAR) on substance abuse and youth in collaboration with WHO in 2001.

(continued)

Table 67. International Support—Kosovo (*Continued*)

UNFPA	▓ Supports PSI's Kosovo Reproductive Health Promotion Project.
	▓ Collaborates with UMCOR on provision of medical and psychosocial counseling and assistance for trafficked people.
UNDP	▓ Information technology and multi-media for information, education and communication.
UNIFEM	▓ Collaborates on several anti-trafficking projects.
	▓ Provides training for lawyers and municipality authorities on gender and local legislation.
WHO	▓ Coordinates TB Commission.
	▓ Chairs Inter-Ministerial Commission on Psychoactive Substances.
	▓ Has supported efforts to undertake HIV surveillance.
	▓ Has seconded a public health coordinator to lead the development and capacity building of Institute for Public Health/Priština.
	▓ With EU, WHO/EURO managing a joint project to rehabilitate blood bank service.
	▓ Participated in rapid appraisal and review (RAR) on substance abuse and youth in Kosovo in collaboration with UNICEF.
UMCOR	▓ Project to increase access to quality sexual health services for bartenders/sex workers. As some women are afforded limited freedom of movement, it was essential to include quality care, such as STI testing and treatment, counselling, and health education, in a secure and private setting as a priority service.
EU CARDS	▓ Assisted development of Kosovo strategy for HIV/AIDS (2004–08).
	▓ Establishment of a policy and planning board and a pharmaceutical unit.
	▓ Implementation of a sustainable telemedicine pilot system.
	▓ Development of a modern and sustainable health information system.
	▓ Establishment of a safe blood transfusion service.
	▓ Support to Priština University's Medical Faculty to raise undergraduate and postgraduate education.
OSCE	▓ Works with IOM, UNMIK Civilian Police (CIVPOL) Trafficking and Prostitution Investigation Units, and UMCOR to protect trafficked person.
	▓ Runs Kosovo Police Service School.
CIDA	▓ Southern Europe HIV/AIDS Prevention/Child Rights: 2001–2004.
	▓ Strengthening Public Health Functions in Balkans: Nov. 2001–June 2004.
	▓ Supports protection and assistance for trafficking victims, including UMCOR's anti-trafficking activities.
USAID	▓ Assisted MOH developing Kosovo strategy for HIV/AIDS.
	▓ Finance HIV-related activities through Save the Children and PSI.
	▓ Supports protection and assistance for trafficking victims.
	▓ Special Initiatives and Cross-Cutting Programs (FY 04 US$6 million): Special initiatives are implemented in health, anti-trafficking and energy. Cross-cutting programs include a women's leadership training activity and a participant training project.

UNTG

The UNTG on HIV/AIDS, which was established in December 2000, has played a crucial role in the coordinated response to HIV/AIDS, especially in the establishment of the Kosovo AIDS Committee and HIV/AIDS Office in the Ministry of Health. The UNTG was initiated by the WHO Office in Kosovo and has been strongly supported by UNICEF, UNFPA and UNDP.

The World Bank is preparing the Kosovo Youth Project to be financed by a grant, and which is expected to include Youth-Friendly Services that will carry out HIV/AIDS prevention activities.

APPENDIX

Table 68. Epidemiological Situation in the Western Balkans

	Albania	Bosnia and Herzegovina	Macedonia	Serbia	Montenegro	Kosovo
HIV cases officially reported 2004	148	101	69	1,921	65	61
AIDS prevalence 2004	<0.1	<0.1	>0.1	<0.1	>0.1	<0.1
Modes of transmission 2004	66% Heterosexual, 10.4% MSM 1.9% MTCT 0.94% IDU	Heterosexual 54% MSM 15% IDU 14%	65% heterosexual 14% MSM 11% IDU 5% MTCT	Heterosexual 24% MSM 30% IDU 14%	50% Heterosexual 25% homosexual	NA
Other STIs officially notified cases	Gonorrhea—6 Syphilis—10 (2000)	Syphilis: 2001—50 2002—25 2003—25 Gonorrhea: Since 1998 ~50 annually	Syphilis—17 Gonorrhea—144	Syphilis: 1,232 (1992–2003) Gonorrhea: 5,231 (1992–2003)	Syphilis—19 (1990–2002) Gonorrhea—181 (1990–2002)	All STI—2,093 (1990–2004)
TB notification rate 2004	18	64	32 109 among refugees 143 in prisons	37	NA	48

Table 69. Vulnerable Groups in the Western Balkans

Vulnerable groups	Albania	Bosnia and Herzegovina	Macedonia	Serbia	Montenegro	Kosovo
Youth	60% under 34 unemployed	Aging population	45% under 30 unemployed	20% under age 15	20% between 15–24	57% of population under 25
	61% teenagers between 14–17 do not attend school	Majority of young people prefer not to use condoms	40% with 2–5 sex partners per year		56% students refer multiple partners	Enrolment in secondary education 55%
	15,000 abandoned children		75% of infected between 20–39		50% refer using condoms	50% refer using condoms for contraception
	Over 30,000 IDUs					
Injecting Drug Users (IDUs)	Mean age <21	6,000–10,000	12,000–15,000	100,000	Mean age 19	Over 5,000
	10–12% of IDU among school children	Mean age when first used drugs 15.4	70% share needles	62% do not consider drug use to be risk factor	67% have 2–5 sex partners per year	Key transit route of heroin into Europe
	13% are CSW	62% do not consider drug use to be risk factor	51% have 2–5 sex partners per year	57% share needles	Relatively low incidence of IDU and needle sharing	Injecting drugs is increasing among youth
	73% share needles	70% do not consider to be at risk of HIV/AIDS	8% are CSW	30% never use condoms	Expected increases in IDU with increased tourist influx	Sharing of needles high
	47% have 2–5 partners per year	70% share needles	88% "never" or "sometimes" use condoms	34% tested for HIV	14% of drugs are bought through CSW	
	85% "never" or only "sometimes" use condoms	50% tested for HIV	96% of IDU-s never tested for HIV	37% positive for Hepatitis C		
	20% tested for HIV	37% Hepatitis C+				
	65% Hepatitis B +					
	18% Hepatitis C +					

(continued)

Table 69. Vulnerable Groups in the Western Balkans (*Continued*)

Vulnerable groups	Albania	Bosnia and Herzegovina	Macedonia	Serbia	Montenegro	Kosovo
Commercial Sex Workers (CSWs)	Over 30,000 30,000 work abroad 62% gave more than 50 partners per year 88% "never" or "sometimes" use condoms Clients pay more to have sex without condoms	11,000–15,000 84% understand that they have increased risk 35% "never" or only "sometimes" use condoms 65 % use drugs 98% have been tested for HIV	5,000–6,000 No information on KAP	3,000 57% use drugs 99% had sex under the influence of drugs 60% use condoms Clients pay more to have sex without condoms 51% tested for HIV	NA	Over 2,000 Most originate from Moldova and Romania, which have higher HIV incidence
Men who have sex with men (MSM)	15–28% of male HIV/AIDS cases	77% use drugs 96% have sex under the influence of drugs 10% tested for HIV	30% have 5–12 sex partners per year 27% engage in group sex 58% never use condoms	58% have more than 2 partners/year 61% always used condoms 77% use drugs 41% tested for HIV	NA	NA
Migrants Refugees IDPs International troops and workers Prisoners Sailors Tourist workers	Migration rate 1% Over 70% HIV cases among young men who contracted the disease abroad 14% victims of trafficking in Italy are Albanian	>250,000 IDPs in Bosnia and Herzegovina >240,000 IDPs in RS 23,500 IDPs in Brcko District 25% working in bars and night clubs are victims of trafficking	25% are seasonal workers. 1,500 prisoners (98% male) 39% IDUs among juvenile prisoners	242,000 IDPs 389,000 refugees	28% HIV infections among sailors and tourist workers Sailors have multiple sexual partners. 6% tested for HIV	300,000 displaced 60,000–70,000 international workers 17,500 international troops

Table 70. National Response to HIV/AIDS in the Western Balkans

	Albania	Bosnia and Herzegovina	Macedonia	Serbia	Montenegro	Kosovo
Intersectoral Coordination	National HIV/AIDS Committee GFATM Country Coordination Mechanism (CCM) appears to be ineffective	National HIV/AIDS Committee	National HIV/AIDS Committee Country Coordination Mechanism Inter-Ministerial Commission to Combat Human Trafficking	Republican AIDS Commission Country Coordination mechanism	Republican AIDS Commission Commission on Substance Abuse	AIDS Committee Inter-ministerial Group for Anti-trafficking Issues Inter-ministerial Commission for Psychoactive Substances
National HIV/AIDS Strategy and Legislation	AIDS Strategy approved Law on AIDS Prevention approved National AIDS Program developed Law on Blood Transfusion approved Law on Reproductive Health under discussion in the Parliament	AIDS Strategy approved National Plan for Action to combat trafficking approved in 2001 GFATM grant proposal was not accepted. A revised application will be submitted.	AIDS Strategy approved Agreement on Prevention and Combating Trans-border Crime ratified Protocol re. Trafficking of People has been signed GFATM grant proposal approved	Strategic Plan prepared but not yet approved GFATM grant proposal approved	Action Plan for Drug Abuse Prevention developed in 2001, but not yet implemented GFATM grant proposal was not accepted. A revised application will be submitted.	AIDS Strategy (2004–2008) approved HIV/AIDS Action Plan issued in 2001 Health Policy Guidelines include HIV/AIDS GFATM grant proposal was not accepted. A revised application will be submitted.

(continued)

Table 70. National Response to HIV/AIDS in the Western Balkans (*Continued*)

	Albania	Bosnia and Herzegovina	Macedonia	Serbia	Montenegro	Kosovo
Government institutions responsible for HIV/AIDS	National HIV/AIDS Committee chaired by the Vice-Prime Minister rarely meets The Institute of Public Health (IPH) leads the National Program for HIV/AIDS. National AIDS Program until recently was staffed only by 2 people, although the government recently allocated funds to enlarge activities	Ministry of Civil Affairs chairs National Advisory Board for Action against HIV/AIDS Institute of Public Health collects epidemiological data on HIV/AIDS	National AIDS Committee under MOH Republican Institute of Health Protection in Skopje is the central institution for public health. Has 10 regional Institutes and 21 branch offices Clinic for Infectious Diseases, Institute of Clinical Biochemistry, Republic Institute for Health Protection, Institute of Transfusion provide testing The Institute of Transfusion ensures national coordination of blood donation.	Republic AIDS Commission is undertaking strategic planning process. Institute of Public Health collects epidemiological data on HIV/AIDS HIV testing (also available at regional IPHs)	The Republican AIDS Commission has been established (RCA), which seeks to address HIV/AIDS in a multisectoral fashion, and works closely with the UN-TG The Republican Institute of Public Health (IPH) has statutory responsibility over prevention and surveillance of HIV/AIDS and STIs 21 District Primary Health Centers (PHC) report HIV/AIDS cases to IPH	Kosovo AIDS Committee (KAC) established Institute for Public Health (IPH) in Pristina conducted KAP survey All HIV infections are reported to IPH

Table 71. HIV/AIDS Prevention and Treatment in the Western Balkans

	Albania	Bosnia and Herzegovina	Macedonia	Serbia	Montenegro	Kosovo
Surveillance	Surveillance System monitors HIV/AIDS, but there has been no sero-prevalence survey. No systematic HIV sentinel surveillance	Integrated system of routine surveillance is not available.	Low reporting of STIs, low number of registered IDUs and other deficiencies in the system suggest serious weaknesses of the surveillance system	22 district IPHs report to the Republican Institute of Public Health in Belgrade	IPH has responsibility over surveillance Integrated system of routine surveillance is not available.	The system is very weak but emphasis is placed on high-risk groups Sentinel sites for HIV/AIDS established but functioning poorly
Notification	Data sent through the District Epidemiological Services at a local level to the IPH	Data from cantonal level is collected by Federal Institute of Public Health of Bosnia and Herzegovina and by IPF for Republika Sprska (RS)	Roles and responsibilities of different institutions in reporting are not well defined.	Notification is done at cantonal levels using preprinted report form.	Many public health laboratory-confirmed STI cases are not reported, and there are reporting delays	The National IPH receives information on all registered HIV/AIDS cases
Testing and counseling	12 testing centers in Tirana, and 12 prefecture blood centers are responsible for routine blood screening Voluntary testing free of charge	Testing is available in several transfusion centers in FBiH and RS. Positive samples are sent to central laboratories in Sarajevo and Belgrade for confirmation	Testing available at 4 public facilities and a few private clinics in Skopje Testing costs €20 without doctor's referral	Testing available in transfusion centers for blood donors, and IPHs and Student Clinics Positive samples sent to central laboratories in Belgrade for confirmation	Anonymous testing illegal and unavailable No allocation of funding for HIV/AIDS testing in MOH and Health Insurance Fund	No formal program available except for international troops Voluntary HIV tests offered but recognized standards are not met

(continued)

Table 71. HIV/AIDS Prevention and Treatment in the Western Balkans (*Continued*)

	Albania	Bosnia and Herzegovina	Macedonia	Serbia	Montenegro	Kosovo
Blood Safety	Law on Blood Transfusion passed in 1995, but remunerated blood donation continues 7.1% of donated blood in 2001 was infected	Free testing for HIV is offered to all blood donors	All donated blood products undergo mandatory testing for HIV 48,000–50,000 blood units tested each year	Free testing for HIV is offered to all blood donors	All donated blood is screened using rapid test methods Four HIV+ samples have been identified	Blood donors tested for HIV, syphilis and Hepatitis B and C Blood donated mostly from extended family members
Condoms	74% of men consider condom price reasonable UNFPA provides condoms	PSI/Risknet provide condoms Vulnerable groups targeted	PSI/Risknet provide condoms	Limited condom distribution is done by NGOs and government clinics	No free provision IDUs report not using condoms because of cost	Local NGOs provide condoms
Prevention	Preventive activities are undertaken mostly by NGOs Most preventive services located in Tirana	Preventive activities are undertaken mostly by NGOs	Preventive activities are undertaken mostly by NGOs but GFATM funding may change the situation	Preventive activities are undertaken mostly by NGOs but GFATM funding may change the situation	No allocation of funding for HIV/AIDS prevention in MOH and HIF	HIV/AIDS prevention included in 5 year strategic plan prepared by KAC and MOH
Treatment	The Tirana University Hospital Center (TUHC) treats most infected patients	Four Clinics of Infectious disease in FBiH offer treatment Guidelines for ART are being developed	The Health Insurance Fund pays for drugs. However, only five patients were being treated	The Clinical University Center, Belgrade provides treatment for 500 patients, including 300 on ARVs	Patients are referred to the Clinical University Center in Belgrade	HIV/AIDS patients are treated at the University Clinical Center in Pristina

References

AbouZahr, C., and T., Wardlaw. 2003. *Maternal Mortality in 2000: Estimates developed by WHO, UNICEF and UNFPA*. Geneva: WHO and UNICEF.

Albania. 2004. "Scaling up the National Response to HIV/AIDS and Tuberculosis." GFATM draft proposal.

Amnesty International. 2003. *Bosnia and Herzegovina: Shelving Justice: War Crimes Prosecutions in Paralysis*. Sarajevo.

Archibald, C. 2002. *Rapid Assessment of Macedonia HIV/AIDS/STI Surveillance System*. Ottawa: Health Canada.

———. 2003. *Rapid Assessment of HIV/AIDS/STI Surveillance System of Bosnia-Herzegovina*. Ottawa: Health Canada.

Ástgeirsdóttir, K. 2001. "Women and Girls in Kosovo: The Effects of Armed Conflict on the Lives of Women." In *The Impact of Armed Conflict on Women and Girls: A Consultative Meeting on Mainstreaming Gender in Areas of Conflict and Reconstruction*. Bratislava.

Baran, O. 2002. UNICEF/OSI Regional Proceedings to the Action Plan Workshop, Sarajevo, February 11–13.

Barnett, T., and A. Whiteside. 2002. *AIDS in the Twenty-first Century: Disease and Globalization*. London: Palgrave Publications.

Bernd, R., and M. McKee. 2003. *Healing the Crises: A prescription for Public Health Action in South Eastern Europe*. Open Society Institute.

Bjekic, M. 2000. "Incidence of Early Syphilis in Belgrade, 1985–1999." *CEEDVA* 2:5–9.

———. 2003. "Prevencija I kontriola seksulano prenosivih infekcija I hepatitisa: analiza odgovora." Report in Serbian for the Global Fund Against AIDS, TB and Malaria.

Bjekic, M., G. Isailovic, and A. Bogavas. 1999. "Pediclosis pubis-udruzenost with other sexually transmitted disease" (in Serbian). *Acta Infectologica Yugoslavica* 4:109–114.

Bjekic, M., H. Vlajinac, and S. Sipetic. 1998. "Demografske karakteristike obolelih od gonoreje u Beogradu u periodu od 1988. do 1994. godine" (in Serbian). *Vojonsant Pregl* 55:289.

Bonnel, R. 2000. *Economic Analysis of HIV/AIDS*. Washington, D.C.: The World Bank.

———. FYRO Macedonia: Proposal to the GFATM.

Bosnia and Herzegovina AIDS Commission 2003. "Bosnia and Herzegovina Strategy on Prevention and Fight Against HIV/AIDS."

Bosnia and Herzegovina Council of Ministers/Ministry of Foreign Trade and Economic Relations/Office of the Bosnia and Herzegovina Coordinator for PRSP. 2003. "Development Strategy of Bosina and Herzegovina (2003–2007): Poverty Reduction Strategy Paper." Second draft for public discussion. Sarajevo.

Cain, J, and Jakubowski (editors). 2002. *Bosnia and Herzegovina, Health Care Systems in Transition*. Copenhagen: European Observatory on Health Care Systems.

Cava, G., and others. 2004. "Young People in South East Europe: From Risk to Empowerment." Discussion Draft. The World Bank.

———. 2005. "Approach Paper : Mainstreaming Youth Issues in ECA." ECSSD, The World Bank.

Clert, C., and others 2004. "Human Trafficking in South Eastern Europe: Beyond Crime Control, An Agenda for Social Inclusion and Development." Internal Draft. The World Bank.

Cucic, V., V. Bjegovic, I. Ignjatovic-Ristic, B. Ilic, and V. Beara. 2002. *Rapid Assessment and Response on HIV/AIDS Among Especially Vulnerable Young People in Serbia*. Belgrade: UNICEF.

Doctors of the World/USA. 2002. "Maternal and Infant Health Project: 1998–2002: Final Report." Pristina.

DFID. 2002. *Southeastern Europe Conference on HIV/AIDS: Implementing the Global Declaration Of Commitment On HIV/AIDS*. Bucharest, Romania: USAID.

EC and The World Bank 2003. Economic Reconstruction and Development in South East Europe. Information about Kosovo. Accessed December. Brussels.

EuroHIV, 2003. *HIV/AIDS Surveillance in Europe: Mid-Year Report 2003*. European Centre for the Epidemiological Monitoring of AIDS, European HIV/AIDS Surveillance Network. Saint-Maurice: Institut de Veille Sanitaire.

EuropeAid (EC Cooperation Office) 2003a. *Annual Action Programme 2003 for Kosovo*. Brussels.

———. 2003b. *Case Study: Supporting Civil Society and Media (Kosovo)*. Brussels.

European Observatory on Health Care Systems. 2002. *Health Care Systems in Transition Summary: The Former Yugoslav Republic of Macedonia*. Copenhagen.

European Union. 2003. *The EU's Relations with South Eastern Europe: Bosnia and Herzegovina: Commission Approves Feasibility Study*. Brussels.

Felzer, S. 2004. *Public Opinion Research: Attitudes Towards HIV/AIDS in Albania: Developing a Strategy to Support Prevention Efforts*. Washington D.C.: The World Bank.

Ferizi, M. 2003. *Epidemiology and Diagnosis of STI Among Young People in Kosovo*. Pristina: Medical Faculty. Available only in Albanian.

Gilgen, D., and others. 2002. "Impact of Organized Violence on Illness Experience of Turkish/Kurdish and Bosnian Migrant Patients in Primary Care." *J Travel Med* 9(5):236–40.

Global Fund to Fight AIDS, Tuberculosis and Malaria (GFATM). 2003a. Portfolio of Grants in Macedonia FYR. Accessed December 2003. Geneva.

———. 2003b. Portfolio of Grants in Serbia. Accessed December. Geneva.

Godinho, J., T. Novotny, H. Tadesse, and A. Vinokur. 2004. *HIV/AIDS and Tuberculosis in Central Asia: Country Profiles*. World Bank Working Paper No. 20. Washington, D.C.: The World Bank.

Godinho, J., A. Renton, V. Vinogradov, T. Novotny, M.J. Rivers, G. Gotsadze, and M. Bravo. 2005. *Reversing the Tide: Priorities for HIV/AIDS Prevention in Central Asia*. World Bank Working Paper No. 54. Washington, D.C.: The World Bank.

Goodson, J. 2003. "Socio-Cultural Aspects of Sexual and Reproductive Health in Kosovo." *Entre Nous: The European Magazine for Sexual and Reproductive Health* (55), UNFPA and WHO.

Gotsadze, T., M. Chawla, and K. Chkatarashvili. 2003. *HIV/AIDS in Georgia*. World Bank Working Paper No. 23. Washington, D.C.: The World Bank.

Government of the Republic of Macedonia. 2000. Interim Poverty Reduction Strategy Paper. Skopje.

Government of the Republic of Montenegro. 2002. Interim Poverty Reduction Strategy Paper. Podgorica.

Government of the Republic of Serbia. 2003. Poverty Reduction Strategy Paper for Serbia. Belgrade.

Grund, J. 2001. "A candle Lit from Both Sides: The Epidemic of HIV Infection in Central and Eastern Europe." In K. McElrath (ed.), *HIV and AIDS: A Global View*.

Hamers, F., and F. Downs. 2003. "HIV in Central and Eastern Europe." *Lancet* 361(9362): 1035–44.

Homans, H. 2003. *Mapping Report: Youth Friendly Services in Bosnia and Herzegovina*. WHO/UNICEF/UNFPA.

Human Rights Watch. 2002. *Hopes Betrayed: Trafficking of Women and Girls to Post-Conflict Bosnia and Herzegovina for Forced Prostitution*. New York.

International Centre for Migration and Health (ICMH) in collaboration with the Albanian Institute of Public Health and coordinated by UNICEF/Albania. 2000. *Knowledge, Attitudes, Practices and Beliefs Survey: Reproductive and Family Health Related Issues in Albania*. Tirana.

International Committee of the Red Cross. 2003. *News: Bosnia and Herzegovina: New Progress on the Missing*. Sarajevo.

International Crisis Group Balkans. 2002. *Macedonia's Public Secret: How Corruption Drags the Country Down*. Skopje/Brussels.

International Organization for Migration (IOM). 2003. "Iraq, Bosnia and Herzegovina." IOM press briefing notes, Sarajevo, October 3.

International Organization for Migration and UNICEF. 2002. *Overview of HIV/AIDS in South Eastern Europe*. Rome

International Planned Parenthood Federation. 2003. http://ippfnet.ippf.org/pub/ IPPF_Regions/IPPF_CountryProfile.asp?ISOCode=AL#Sexual

Institute of Public Health (IPH) of the Federation of Bosnia and Herzegovina, and Ministry of Health and Social Welfare of Republika Srpska. 2002. "Household Survey of Women and Children: Bosnia-Herzegovina 2000: A Multiple Indicator Cluster Survey." Draft Final Report. Sarajevo: UNICEF.

Kakarriqi, E.Z. 2003. *Epidemiological Background of Infectious Diseases in Albania (1960–2001) and Their Prevention and Control in the Context of Natural Disasters and Infectious Diseases*. Tirana: ILAR

Kovacs, L. 1997. "Abortion and Contraceptive Practices in Eastern Europe." *International Journal of Gynecology and Obstetrics* 58:69–75.

Kulis, M., M. Chawla, A. Kozierkiewicz, and E. Subata. 2003. *Truck Drivers and Casual Sex: An Inquiry Into the Potential Spread of HIV/AIDS in the Baltic Region*. World Bank Working Paper No. 37. Washington, D.C.: the World Bank.

Leimanowska, B. 2002. *Trafficking in Human Beings in Southeastern Europe-Current Situation and Responses*. Belgrade: UNICEF, Area Office for the Balkans.

Lundberg, M. 2001. "Economic Analysis. Moldova AIDS Control Project Appraisal Document, and Belarus TB/AIDS Control Project Appraisal Document." Washington, D.C.: The World Bank.

Macedonia Country Coordinating Mechanism (CCM). 2003. "Proposal to the Global Fund to Fight AIDS, TB and Malaria: Round 3: Building a Coordinated National Response to Tuberculosis and HIV/AIDS in Macedonia." Skopje.

Macedonian Interethnic Association (MIA). 2002. *KAPB Survey Among Women of Reproductive Age in R. Macedonia.*

Macedonia National Multisectoral HIV/AIDS Commission. 2003. *Macedonia HIV/AIDS National Strategy 2003–2006.* Skopje.

Mahmutovic, S., E. Beslagic, M. Seremet, and S. Cavaljuga. 2003. "Diagnosis of Chlamydial Infections—Personal Experience." *Med Arh* 573:137–40. Abstract only.

Miller, D., and A. Ryskulova. 2004. *Surveillance Systems in Eastern Europe and Central Asia.* Washington D.C.: The World Bank.

Ministry of Health of Serbia. 2003. *Better Health for All in the Third Millennium: Health Policy, Vision and Strategy 2003–2015.* Belgrade. Serbian only.

Momartin, S. and others. 2003. "Dimensions of Trauma Associated with Posttraumatic Stress Disorder (PTSD) Caseness, Severity and Functional Impairment: A Study of Bosnian Refugees Resettled in Australia." *Soc Sci Med* 57(5):775–81.

North Atlantic Treaty Organization (NATO). 2003. *SFOR Plans Future Force Structure.* Brussels.

Novotny, T., D. Haazen, and O. Adeyi. 2003. *HIV/AIDS in Southeastern Europe: Case Studies from Bulgaria, Croatia, and Romania.* World Bank Working Paper No. 4. Washington D.C.: The World Bank.

Office of the United Nations High Commissioner for Human Rights. 2003. *Annual Appeal 2004: Overview of Activities and Financial Requirements.* Geneva.

Open Society Institute. 2003. Open Society Fund–Bosnia and Herzegovina. Accessed December 2003. New York: Open Society Institute.

Population Reference Bureau (PRB). 2003. *World Population Data Sheet 2003.* Washington, D.C.

Population Services International. 2003. *Drug Risk Reduction.* Washington, D.C.

Refugees International. 2003a. *Country Information: Albania.* Washington, D.C.

———. 2003b. *Country Information: Kosovo.* Washington, D.C.

Republic of Albania National Committee of Women and Family and UNICEF. 2000. *Mapping of Existing Information on Domestic Violence in Albania.* Tirana.

Republic of Serbia (Serbia and Montenegro) National Country Coordinating Mechanism for AIDS and TB. 2003. "Proposal to the Global Fund to Fight AIDS, TB and Malaria: Round 3: Control of Tuberculosis in Serbia (Serbia and Montenegro) Through Implementation of DOTS Strategy and Outreach Services for Vulnerable Populations." Belgrade.

Rhodes, T., and others. 2003. *HIV Prevention Priorities for Vulnerable Populations: Key Findings from Consultations with Experts.* London: DFID HIV Prevention Among Vulnerable Populations Initiative in Serbia and Montenegro.

Ringold, D., M. Orenstein, and E. Wilkens. 2003. *Roma in an Expanding Europe: Breaking the Poverty Cycle.* Washington, D.C.: The World Bank.

Ruhel, C., and others. 2002. *The Economic Impact of HIV/AIDS in the Russian Federation.* Moscow: The AIDS Centre/The World Bank.

Sedlecki. 1999. "Promotion of Reproductive Health of Adolescents." Youth Friendly Services in Primary Health Care, Republic Centre for Family Planning, Institute for Mother and Child, Serbia.

Sharp, S. 2004. *Informing Policy Thorugh Modelling: A Case Study of the Socio-Economic Implications of AIDS in Russia.* Gastein: European Health Forum.

Spector, B.I., S. Winbourne, and L.D. Beck. 2003. *Corruption in Kosovo: Observations and Implications for USAID.* Washington, D.C.: USAID and Management Systems International.

Statistical Office of Kosovo. 2003a. *Crimes Reported to the Police.* Pristina.

———. 2003b. *Kosovo and Its Population.* Pristina.

Stevenson, D. 2003. *Serbia and Montenegro Health Profile.* London: DFID Health Systems Resource Centre.

Transparency International. 2003. *Corruption Perceptions Index 2003.* Berlin.

UN Commission on Human Rights. 2003. *Specific Groups and Individuals: Other Vulnerable Groups and Individuals: The Protection of Human Rights in the Context of Human Immunodeficiency Virus (HIV) and Acquired Immune Deficiency Syndrome (AIDS): Report of the Secretary-General.* Geneva.

UN Office on Drugs and Crime. 2002. *Seventh United Nations Survey of Crime Trends and Operations of Criminal Justice Systems, Covering the Period 1998–2000.* Center for International Crime Prevention. Vienna.

———. 2003. *Global Illicit Drug Trends 2003.* Vienna.

UN News Service. 2003. *UN Transfers Final Government Responsibilities to Kosovo Institutions.* Geneva.

UN Security Council. 2003. *Bosnia: Monthly Report to the UN on the Operations of the Stabilization Force.* New York.

UNAIDS. 2001a. *Assisted Response to HIV/AIDS, STIs and Drug Abuse in Central Asian Countries 1996–2000.* Geneva: UNAIDS.

———. 2001b. UNAIDS Joint Mission on HIV/AIDS and Peacekeeping. UNMIK and UNMIBH (UNAIDS, UNFPA, DPKO), Pristina, November 19–21; Sarajevo, November 22–24. Geneva.

———. 2002a. *AIDS Epidemic Update.* Geneva.

———. 2002b. *Epidemiological Fact Sheets on HIV/AIDS and STI, Albania.* 2002 Update.

———. 2002c. *Epidemiological Fact Sheets on HIV/AIDS and STI, Bosnia and Herzegovina.* 2002 Update.

———. 2002d. *Epidemiological Fact Sheets on HIV/AIDS and STI, The Former Yugoslav Republic of Macedonia.* 2002 Update.

———. 2002e. *Epidemiological Fact Sheets on HIV/AIDS and STI, Yugoslavia.* 2002 Update.

———. 2002f. "HIV/AIDS in South Eastern Europe—The Regional Situation." Proceedings of the Conference on HIV/AIDS in SEE. Bucharest.

———. 2002g. *Macedonia: Epidemiological Fact Sheet on HIV/AIDS and Sexually Transmitted Infections: 2002 Update.* Geneva.

———. 2002h. *Report on the Global HIV/AIDS Epidemic.* Geneva.

———. 2003a. *AIDS Epidemic Update.* Geneva.

————. 2003b. *Follow-up to the 2001 United Nations General Assembly Special Session on HIV/AIDS: Progress Report on the Global Response to the HIV/AIDS Epidemic, 2003.* Geneva.

————. 2003c. *On the Front Line: A Review of Policies and Programmes to Address HIV/AIDS Among Peacekeepers and Uniformed Services.* Geneva.

————. 2003d. *Serbia and Montenegro: Follow-up to the Declaration of Commitment on HIV/AIDS (UNGASS). Reporting period: January-December 2002.* Annex 2: National Composite Policy Index Questionnaire. Geneva.

————. 2003e. "Albania Country Fact Sheet." Accessed November. Geneva.

UNAIDS and WHO. 2000. "AIDS Epidemic Explodes in Eastern Europe." Press Release. Berlin: UNAIDS/WHO.

UNAIDS and The World Bank. 2003. *Funding Requirements for the response to HIV/AIDS in ECA.*

UNDP. 2002. Preventive Development Advocacy on HIV/AIDS in Kosovo. http://www. kosovo.undp.org/Projects/HIV/hiv.htm.

————. 2003. *Human Development Report 2003.* New York.

UNFPA. 2003a. *State of World Population 2003.* Secretariat/Department of Economic and Social Affairs/Population Division. New York.

————. 2003b. *Profile: Kosovo.* Pristina.

UNFPA and Population Reference Bureau (PRB). 2003. *Country Profiles for Population and Reproductive Health: Policy Developments and Indicators 2003.* New York.

UNICEF. 2000. *Multiple Indicator Cluster Survey Report: Albania.* Tirana.

————. 2001. *Multiple Indicator Cluster Survey II: The Report for the Federal Republic of Yugoslavia.* Belgrade.

————. 2002a. *Rapid Assessment of HIV/AIDS/STI Surveillance System of FYR Serbia.*

————. 2002b. *Rapid Assessment of HIV/AIDS/STI Surveillance System of FYR Macedonia.*

————. 2002c. *Rapid Assessment and Response on HIV/AIDS Among Especially Vulnerable Young People in Albania.* Tirana.

————. 2003a. At A Glance: Serbia and Montenegro. Accessed Decembe.

————. 2003b. Information by Country: The Former Yugoslav Republic of Macedonia. Accessed December. New York.

————. 2003c. *Social Monitor 2003: CEE/CIS/Baltic States.* Innocenti Research Centre, Florence.

United Nations. 2002a. *Abortion Policies: A Global Review.* Population Division/Department of Economic and Social Affairs. New York.

————. 2002b. *The Albanian Response to the Millennium Development Goals.* Prepared by Human Development Promotion Center (HDPC).

————. 2003. *World Population Prospects: The 2002 Revision: Highlights.* Secretariat/ Department of Economic and Social Affairs/Population Division. New York.

USAID. 2002. *HIV/AIDS Prevention in Kosovo.*

U.S. Department of State. 2003a. *Background Notes: Albania.* Washington, D.C.

————. 2003b. *Background Note: Bosnia and Herzegovina.* Washington, D.C.

————. 2003c. *Background Notes: Serbia and Montenegro.* Washington, D.C.

————. 2003d. *Background Notes: The Former Yugoslav Republic of Macedonia.* Washington, D.C.

————. 2003e. *Victims of Trafficking and Violence Protection Act of 2000: Trafficking in Persons Report*. Washington, D.C.

Wennberg, J.L., and X. Jakupi. 2002. "Prevalence of HIV in TB Patients in Kosovo." Abstract no. ThPeC7556. in *XIV International AIDS Conference*. Barcelona.

WHO. 2001. "Review of the Information from Operational Research and Socio-Behavioural Surveys on Sexual Behaviour and Condom Use in Eastern Europe and Central Asia." Prepared by I. Eramova and I. Toskin.

————. 2002. *DOTS Expansion Plan to Stop TB in the WHO European Region 2002–2006*. Copenhagen.

————. 2003. *Global Tuberculosis Control: Surveillance, Planning, Financing*. Geneva.

Wong, E. 2002a. *Rapid Assessment and Response on HIV/AIDS Among Especially Vulnerable Young People in South Eastern Europe*. Belgrade: UNICEF.

————. 2002b. *Rapid Assessment of Montenegro HIV/AIDS/STI Surveillance System. Field Investigation Report, September 28–October 2, 2002*.

————. 2002c. *Rapid Assessment of Serbia HIV/AIDS/STI Surveillance System: Field Investigation Report: September 25–28, 2002 (revised)*. Ottawa: Health Canada, Centre for Infectious Disease Prevention and Control.

World Bank. 2000. "Country Assistance Strategy: Bosnia and Herzegovina." Europe and Central Asia Region/South East Europe Country Unit. Washington, D.C.

————. 2001. "Kosovo: Poverty Assessment: Volume 1: Main Report." Europe and Central Asia Region/Poverty Reduction and Economic Management Unit. Washington, D.C.

————. 2002a. "Country Assistance Strategy Progress Report: Bosnia and Herzegovina." Europe and Central Asia Region/South East Europe Country Unit Washington, D.C.

————. 2002b. "Country Brief: Kosovo." Washington, D.C.

————. 2002c. "Federal Republic of Yugoslavia: Legal and Judicial Diagnostic." Legal Department. Washington, D.C.: World Bank.

————. 2002d. "Public Expenditure and Institutional Review."

————. 2002e. "Serbia Public Expenditures Review."

————. 2003a. *Averting AIDS Crises in Eastern Europe and Central Asia*. Washington D.C.: The World Bank.

————. 2003b. "Bosnia and Herzegovina Country Brief 2003." Washington, D.C.

————. 2003c. "Bosnia and Herzegovina: Projects and Reports." Washington, D.C.

————. 2003d. "Country Assistance Strategy for The Former Yugoslav Republic of Macedonia." Washington, D.C.

————. 2003e. "Country Brief: Serbia and Montenegro." Washington, D.C.

————. 2003f. "Kosovo: Economic Assistance Grant." Washington, D.C.

————. 2003g. "Serbia and Montenegro-Serbia Health Project." Washington, D.C.

————. 2003h. "Serbia and Montenegro: Poverty Assessment." Europe and Central Asia Region/Poverty Reduction and Economic Management Unit. Washington, D.C.

————. 2003i. *World Development Indicators 2003*. Washington, D.C.

————. 2003j. "Albania Country Brief 2003." Washington, D.C..

————. 2004a. "Poverty Reduction Strategy Paper."

————. 2004b. "Project Information Document: Appraisal Stage:Montenegro Health System Improvement Project." Washington, D.C.

Eco-Audit

Environmental Benefits Statement

The World Bank is committed to preserving Endangered Forests and natural resources. We print World Bank Working Papers and Country Studies on 100 percent postconsumer recycled paper, processed chlorine free. The World Bank has formally agreed to follow the recommended standards for paper usage set by Green Press Initiative—a nonprofit program supporting publishers in using fiber that is not sourced from Endangered Forests. For more information, visit www.greenpressinitiative.org.

In 2004, the printing of these books on recycled paper saved the following:

Trees*	Solid Waste	Water	Net Greenhouse Gases	Electricity
307	14,387	130,496	28,262	52,480
'40' in height and 6-8" in diameter	Pounds	Gallons	Pounds	KWH

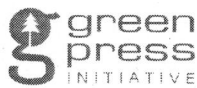

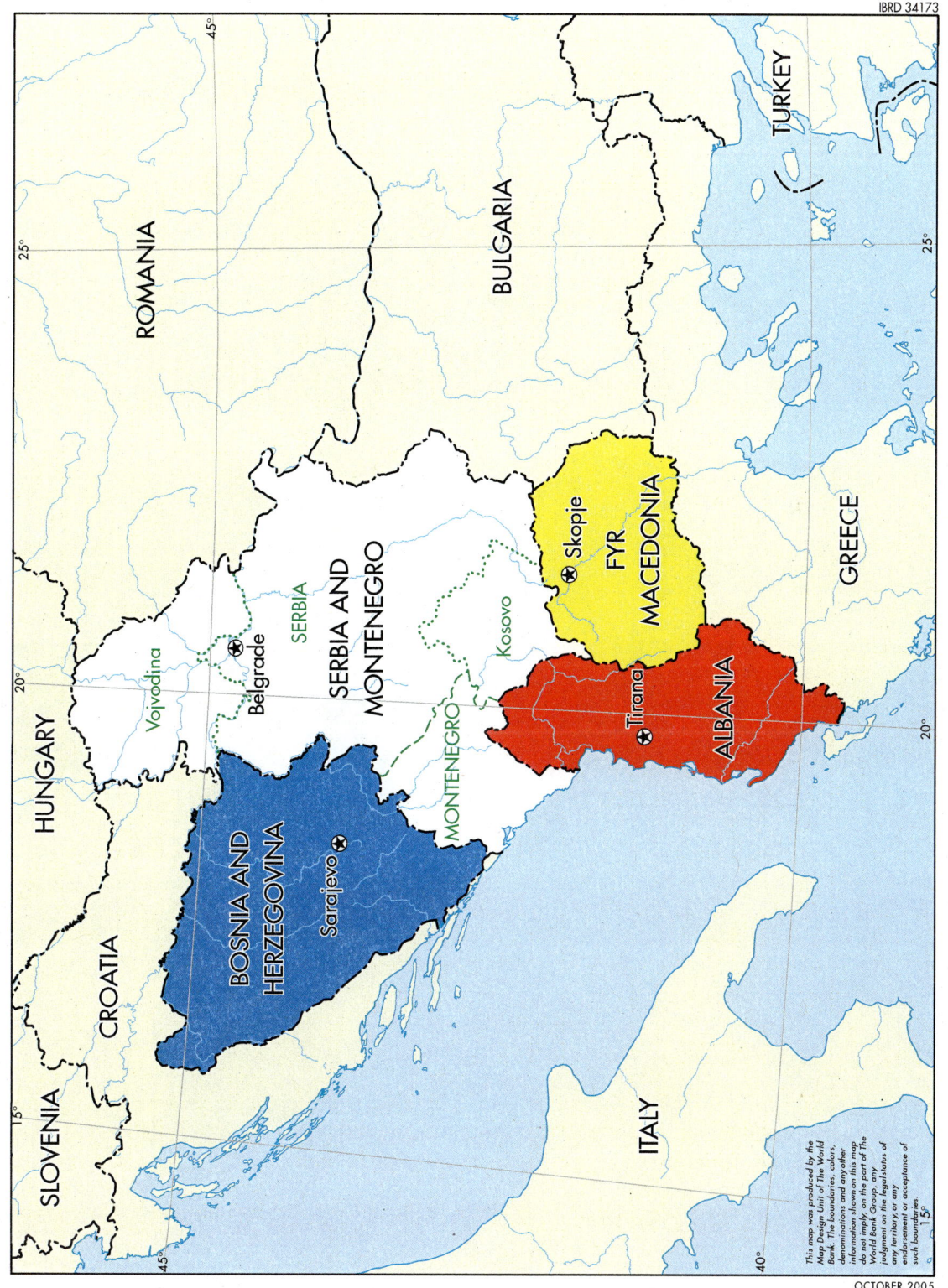

IBRD 34173

OCTOBER 2005

SLOVENIA

CROATIA

HUNGARY

ROMANIA

BULGARIA

TURKEY

GREECE

ITALY

ALBANIA

FYR
MACEDONIA

SERBIA AND
MONTENEGRO

SERBIA

Vojvodina

Kosovo

MONTENEGRO

BOSNIA AND
HERZEGOVINA

Belgrade

Sarajevo

Tirana

Skopje

45°

25°

20°

15°

45°

40°

15°

25°

20°